*Parting Wild H Mane p. 135*
*Retreat step p. 85*

# T'ai-Chi Ch'üan
### (WU STYLE)

Body and Mind in Harmony:
The Integration of Meaning and Method

## by Sophia Delza

*Foreword by Robert C. Neville*
*With Drawings by the Author*
*New Photographs by Lisa Lewicki*

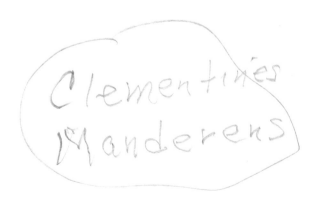

*Clementines*
*Manderens*

**Revised Edition ▪ State University of New York Press**

Published by
State University of New York Press, Albany
Revised Edition 1985
Copyright ©1961 by Sophia Delza
All rights reserved. Cover and text design by Sushila Blackman.
Chinese Calligraphy by Liu Cheng Yü
Library of Congress Cataloging in Publication Data
Delza, Sophia
  T'ai chi ch'üan: body and mind in harmony.

  Bibliography: p.
  Includes index.
  1. T'ai chi ch'üan.   I. Title.   II. Title: Body and
mind in harmony.
GV505.D37      1985        613.7'1        84-23916
ISBN 0-88706-029-3
ISBN 088706-030-7 (pbk.)

10 9

*To Cook A. Glassgold*
*who made it possible for me to live in China*

# Acknowledgements

To Robert C. Neville, Professor of Philosophy and Religious Studies at The State University of New York at Stony Brook, editor of this revised edition, Sophia Delza takes this opportunity to extend her heartfelt gratitude for his extremely invaluable contribution to this book; and deeply appreciates his exceptional patience and perceptive interest at all times. The author will always feel grateful to her teacher in China, Mr. Ma Yüeh-Liang, the grand master of t'ai-chi ch'üan, for having imparted his knowledge to her with such generosity.

She would like particularly to thank Mr. Koo Hsien-Liang, whose scholarly and sensitively artistic translations of Chinese classics helped her immeasurably and who so sympathetically supported her activities.

She is also grateful to Mr. Chang Kuo-Ho, of the United Nations, who suggested that she do the book on T'ai-Chi Ch'üan; the San Francisco T'ai-Chi Ch'üan Club for their warm sponsorship of her performances; Joseph Carter, of the *New York Times*; Nina Gordani for her personal management of the author's performance-lectures; and Hubert Wang, who translated Chinese literature for her.

And especially, the author is happy to acknowledge the honor the members of the United Nations' T'ai- Chi Ch'üan Club have done her by asking her to teach them. There are too many to mention all, but those of the original group are: Hsü Ming-Chen, Djang Chu, Edward Lai, Shih Tao-Tsi, Tsao Hung-Chao, Shen Chang-Jui, Yen Cheng, Wellington Lee (first president), Robert Mok, Booker Lee, and Simon Chang.

# Contents

# Foreword

This book by Sophia Delza presents t'ai-chi ch'üan in two aspects. One is an invitation to understand and try t'ai-chi ch'üan as an exercise, a way of life, with practical personal benefits. The other is an appreciative analysis of the content of the exercise-art as a total structure which succeeds in putting body and mind into harmony— a meaningful goal in China from its earliest times. T'ai-chi ch'üan is a vehicle for bringing many strands of the profound culture of China into our lives, a vehicle for entering some of the formative creations of civilization. In this Foreword I want to focus on the connection between these two aspects.

T'ai-chi ch'üan is usually, and validly, associated with the taoist tradition of China. Yet its root metaphors of yin and yang—presenting the essence of movement or change—are more ancient than taoism and are common to the Confucian and taoist traditions both. It was a Neo-Confucian, Chou Tun-i (Chou Lien-Hsi, 1017-1073 C.E.), who first and most succinctly stated the concepts that unite the practical and historical significance of t'ai-chi ch'üan:

> The Ultimate of Non-being and also the Great Ultimate (T'ai-chi)! The Great Ultimate through movement generates yang. When its activity reaches its limit, it becomes tranquil. Through tranquility the Great Ultimate generates yin. When tranquility reaches its limit, activity begins again. So movement and tranquility alternate and become the root of each other, giving rise to the distinction of yin and yang, and the two modes are thus established.
>
> By the transformation of yang and its union with yin, the Five Agents of Water, Fire, Wood, Metal, and Earth arise. When these five material forces (ch'i) are distributed in harmonious order, the four seasons run their course.[1]

An explication of this historically rooted statement leads to a philosophical understanding of what t'ai-chi ch'üan can do in a practical sense.

Chou's statement expressed the very ancient Chinese ontological sense that insofar as the universe is anything at all (the Great Ultimate, T'ai-chi), it is movement. Movement consists "first" of activity, of extension, of expression. "An" activity has a natural limit which, when reached, deactivates the activity as it were, returning to tranquility. The activity is yang, the tranquility is yin. Or better, being on the way to an activity's limit is yang, returning toward tranquility is yin. Westerners are inclined to believe that there needs to be an actor for there to be activity, and we ask what

---

1. From Chou's "An Explanation of the Diagram of the Great Ultimate," translated by Wing- tsit Chan in his *Source Book in Chinese Philosophy* (Princeton: Princeton University Press, 1963) p. 463.

"it" is that extends toward its limit and returns to base. From this Western perspective it might seem that there are two movements, yang-action and yin-relaxation. But for the Chinese, both yang-action and yin-relaxation to tranquility are required for there to be motion; by themselves, yin and yang are abstractions. There is no actor which moves, only a movement with a definite process, outcome, and shape. Actors as we know them in the large are complex organizations of movements. How can this be? Is it a plausible cosmology?

One element in the metaphoric penumbra of yin is that of the mother, the matrix. I take this to mean that in any situation there is an accumulated product of the past and of the environment.[2] This matrix has a definite shape and set of forces constituting the base from which a novel extension or action is launched. From that richly funded situation an action can commence, and it can extend until it reaches the limits of the resources its matrix situation provides. In human affairs it is possible by artifical means to overextend oneself, running out of resources before one can retreat back to the base of supply. (The *Tao Te Ching* uses military images like this.) A truly natural movement finds its limit at the point where it still has the capacity to return to its matrix, to where its movement is tranquil because it rests in the richly funded and supporting environment.[3] Other metaphoric elements of yin are the low, safe ground, the water which always finds its level and can wear away any rock barring its path. Although yin and yang are always complementary strictly speaking, there is a priority of interest in yin for the Chinese, because yin is both source and fulfillment of action. Were it not for yang, however, nothing would happen. The environment and the past would be barren and there would be no "presence" or spontaneity. Movement requires both active stretching out and the source and point of return for the stretching.

Chou Tun-i described the alternation of yang and yin as a wave: extension and retreat. A wave has amplitude—the distance between crest and trough— and frequency—the number of waves in a given time (or relative to another frequency). Waves therefore can be organized into different patterns, differing by amplitude or frequency. The patterns can be regular for a while, or changing according to changes in amplitutde or frequency. In Chou's view, the basic table of elements, his "Five Agents of Water, Fire, Wood, Metal, and Earth," are constituted by different basic patterns of yang and yin. Although we should be wary about extending the notion of wave patterns or vibratory patterns to the smallest elements

2. This interpretation supports that of Chang Chung-yuan in his brilliant *Creativity and Taoism: A Study of Chinese Philosophy, Art, and Poetry* (New York: Julian Press, 1963; Harper and Row, 1970).
3. I have elaborated this notion of yin-yang movement in *The Tao and the Daimon* (Albany: State University of New York Press, 1982), chapter 7.

our science discovers, it is highly plausible that there is some level of organization of our physical cosmos that has the character of vibratory patterns.[4]

A solid physical object such as a stone is a highly complex harmony of many, many vibratory patterns, a harmony that is relatively stable over time. The solidity of the stone's structure comes from the fact that the component patterns interlock and reinforce one another. They resonate with one another (to introduce a musical metaphor). The harmony in the stone itself depends on support from and tolerance by the patterns of the wider environment: relentless drops of water will wear away a groove, and extreme heat or cold can melt down or crack the integration of vibrations within the rock. Nature is only relatively stable, and a stone endures through changes very slowly. Animals, of course, not only sustain their organic harmony of many wave patterns, but they also change those patterns relative to one another so as to move. More than stones they incorporate patterns originating from outside, metabolize them and excrete the outcomes of the process as new kinds of patterns. More than merely physical changes, the social and emotional lives of higher animals involve participation in super-complex harmonies with other animals and institutions.

The moving universe thus can be conceived as a vast kaleidoscope of shifting wave patterns. Each pattern depends on its environment for tolerance and reinforcement. Patterns change in response to resonances and dissonances with other patterns. Some clusters of vibratory patterns are so organically harmonized that they behave together as an individual; others are more loosely harmonized, as constituting a complex situation. Some patterns may be so remote as to be unaffected by one another except insofar as both are tolerated by the broadest and most basic patterns uniting the universe. Music is a good metaphor for this vision of things. The cosmos is a vast evolving musical composition with many figures and a few themes. There are pockets of intense harmonies and points of shocking dissonance, periods of low grade overall harmony barely able to separate the dischords, and rare moments of high grade harmony where most things seem to reinforce and enrich one another.[5]

The Chinese express the *human* ideal for this vision as "being one body with the world," one body not in the sense of mystical union or physical cohesion but in the sense of resonating sympathetically with all

4. This notion is at the heart of the cosmology of Alfred North Whitehead. See, for instance, his *Science and the Modern World* (New York: Macmillan, 1927), chapter 8, "The Quantum Theory."
5. This musical conception bears resemblance to J.R.R. Tolkien's fantasy, "Ainulindale," in the *Silmarillion* (Boston: Houghton Mifflin, 1977), edited by Christopher Tolkien, except that Tolkien's vision is theistic.

things.[6] Rather than protect our individuality with a thick skin, secure borders of ownership, and an ego that maintains its shape regardless of its circumstance, the Chinese vision, taoist and Confucian alike, is that integrity comes from an openness to things so that we tap and multiply the product of many harmonies. Instead of insulation we need sensitivity and discriminating responsiveness, constantly adjusting our own rhythms in response to the shifting patterns of the universe. Then our own spontaneous actions, the yang elements in our lives, will be empowered by the forces of the universe, by the natural patterns of social, personal, and biological existence. Needless frustration comes from alienating the patterns of others and competing with them. Strength and will are extended by resonating with the rhythms of others and finding the new harmonic patterns of our own which will set up sympathetic responses in others as we want. The Chinese theme of rectifying others by setting them a moral example seems naive from the Western standpoint, and is often ineffective given the barbarous dissonances punctuating human affairs. But from the perspective of the Chinese ontological vision that strategy makes sense. Causation, either close-range or at a distance, consists in setting up a vibratory pattern to which the patterns of other things must conform according to their own matrices.

What does t'ai-chi ch'üan do? It sets up a perfect pattern of movement on the scale of the human body, a pattern with powerful resonating effects both on the sub-patterns within the body and on the larger patterns in which the t'ai-chi player participates. For the twenty or thirty minutes it takes to practice the exercise, one's movements are like a lead singer whose strong voice pulls the other choristers on pitch and establishes the center of the harmony. As the practice proceeds, one's thoughts, emotions, and physiological processes are gradually calmed and brought into synchronization with the tranquilly moving t'ai-chi ch'üan forms. So it is that the practice of t'ai-chi ch'üan is a cultivation of the yin side of life, that part of movement which is returning to tranquility.

It is not being romantic to say that the exercising will greatly reinforce the body's own recuperative powers. It will powerfully help untangle one's own ability to respond, first for a few minutes a day, and then with more carryover throughout life. The effects are felt at the first practice session, and they increase, becoming more pervasive and tangible, as one's skill is honed. This has been the experience of those who have made t'ai-chi ch'üan integral to their lives, and it is what one would expect from the ancient Chinese vision of the cosmos from which it developed.

6. The notion of "being one body with the world" was given its subtlest interpretation by Wang Yang-ming, a 16th Century Neo-Confucianist. See his "Inquiry on the Great Learning," translated by Wing- tsit Chan in his *Source Book*, pp.659-667. I have analyzed Wang's theory in connection with Whitehead's in *The Tao and the Daimon*, chapter 8.

Mastery of t'ai-chi ch'üan not only brings its therapeutic and life-ordering benefits. It also offers a sensuous and direct vehicle for entering into important strands of Chinese experience, strands with extraordinary historical depth. What are the concepts of the Chinese world to us if we have no concrete feel for them? T'ai-chi ch'üan provides exactly such a feel for movement, the fundamental Chinese idea: "The Great Ultimate through movement generates yang. When its activity reaches its limit, it becomes tranquil. Through tranquility the Great Ultimate generates yin. When tranquility reaches its limit, activity begins again."

The causative power of the patterned movements of t'ai-chi ch'üan stems from its innate beauty, its perfection. Perfection of movement and form is what brings the other rhythms into line. The essence of Sophia Delza's presentation of t'ai-chi ch'üan in this book and through her teaching is just that perfection of movement. What this means will be manifest in the text to follow. Here is the place, however, to introduce Sophia Delza herself.

It was no accident that she responded easily to the philosophy and intrinsic perfection of t'ai-chi ch'üan. A native New Yorker, she studied dance, music, and art from an early age, as well as science. Dance became her career and she attained great distinction as a creative dancer and performer, as well as a writer, lecturer, and teacher of the dance-arts. Throughout her many years in Shanghai she studied the Classical Chinese Theatre and especially t'ai-chi ch'üan with Grandmaster Ma Yüeh-Liang, the great living exponent of the *Wu* Chien-Chuan System (*Chia*) of t'ai-chi ch'üan. She devoted herself to his teaching and with her extraordinary preparation in the dance-arts became an understanding and perfect pupil. On her return to the United States she toured extensively, giving lecture-demonstrations and recitals of the Classical Chinese Theatre along with lecture-demonstrations of t'ai-chi ch'üan—the first to do so in America. Her writings on aesthetics, dance-theatre arts, exercise and health have been published in China, Europe and in many journals in the United States, among which are: The Journal of Aesthetics and Art Criticism, Asian Music, Dance Observer, Dynamis, Theatre Drama Review and Chinoperl Papers. Her Record-Album, teaching T'ai-Chi Ch'üan, was issued by Columbia Pictures; a Modern Dance Exercise Book by Hawthorne Books, Inc.; her T'ai-Chi Ch'üan book by Editions Denoël in Paris. She has conducted regular classes at universities, dance institutes, and at the New York Actors' Studio. For many years she has been teaching for the United Nations T'ai-Chi Ch'üan Club which was formed and given a charter when she was asked to teach there. Among other awards she has been inducted into the Hall of Fame of Hunter College. Currently she is teaching at the United Nations, also at the State University of New York College at Purchase, Actors' Studio and at her long established School of T'ai-Chi Ch'üan at Carnegie Hall, where I have studied for a decade.

The first edition of this book, published in 1961, was the earliest presentation of t'ai-chi ch'üan ever to be written by a Westerner. That material has been thoroughly revised and expanded to comprise this new volume, a comprehensive analysis of the exercise-art. In addition to the historical and conceptual introduction and descriptions of the 108 Forms, the greatest original contribution of this new edition is its subtle interpretation of t'ai-chi ch'üan from the standpoint of the balanced harmony of the aesthetic and scientific. Sophia Delza reveals that the ancient exercise-art of t'ai-chi ch'üan is a profound, complex, universal entity which can be mastered by all and which can become a living component of any culture.

It is a great pleasure to introduce this entryway into the world of t'ai-chi ch'üan.

*Robert C. Neville*
*July, 1984*

# THE WAY of the T'AI-CHI CH'ÜAN WAY

The body is alerted at every moment in a quiet way
   With the quiet way, energy is focused in a balanced way
With the balanced way, heart-mind coordinates in a perceptive way
   With perception, action is centered in a unified way
And with unity, mind-body functions in a tranquil way

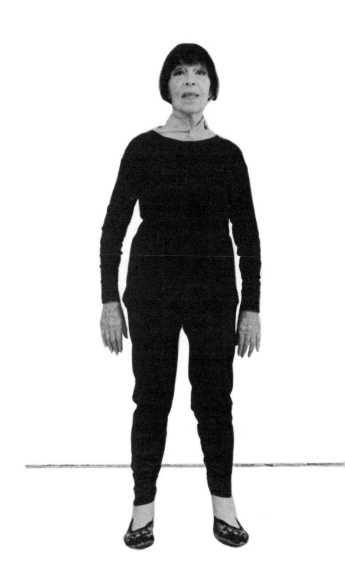

# INTRODUCTION: By Way of a Beginning

*"What is past one cannot amend,*
*For the future one can always provide."*
    —From the *Analects* of Confucius

## A Contemporary View

Is there anyone in the world whose idea of being truly healthy would not include, along with a healthy body, a fine mind combined with an ease of disposition? Fleeting glimpses of this feeling of harmony are experienced by everyone at some time in his or her life. In our colloquialisms we see revealed the clear inner relationship of mind and body. "I feel as if I were floating" is a common expression to describe a peak of physical contentment. Well-being produces a sensation of lightness where the body is sensed but not felt. "I'm simply walking on air" is an image that almost obliterates the body and makes the spirit seem all powerful.

What agony of indecision and what physical immobility are exposed by "I'm all tied up in knots." Similarly, "My heart stood still" expresses anxiety that almost strangles circulation. Composure and mental equilibrium can hardly be sustained in a weak and unhealthy system where discomfort dominates the consciousness.

The effect of body on mind and mind on body is evidenced in every turn of our daily lives. This realization is often a step toward seeking a technique that can "nourish the body and calm the spirit"—that, as an exercise, can give action to thought, and, as a philosophy, can give thought to action, and which as a composite art is so synthesized as to make the whole greater than the sum of its intriguing parts.

The art of exercise, both physical and philosophical, goes far back into China's history, with "mind" as the dominating factor for correct and total body development. The Chinese recognized that our instinctive and mechanical innate movements are not enough to extend life's span or to develop and even to sustain optimal health. Mental motivation and attentively manipulated motion with intricate coordination are necessary to produce inner vitality and outer versatility, both essential for harmonious living.

Such is t'ai-chi ch'üan (pronounced tye gee chwan), the unique Chinese system of Soft-Intrinsic Exercise. Dating back to C.E. 1000, this exercise is extremely popular today. In the present century five major t'ai-chi ch'üan styles (P'ai) are being practiced: Yang, Wu, Ho, Sun, and Chen. This book illustrates the *Wu*, a style that concentrates on harmonious self-development with the philosophical as well as the psychological aspects emphasized. It has as its goal the achievement of health and tranquility by means of a "way of movement": a technique of moving slowly and continuously, without strain, through a varied sequence of contrasting Forms that create stable vitality with calmness, balanced strength with flexibility, controlled energy with awareness.

There is a significant difference in concept between the dance-art that is used as an exercise and the exercise that is an art in itself. As a modern dancer I appreciate this, having created dance forms for the purpose of art and for exercise. Designed movements, patterns, and excerpts of dance techniques, which are extracted from the dance-art for use as general exercise, though inevitably stimulating and enlivening, must be considered inadequate for the more profound, permanent aspect of the development of mind and body.

T'ai-chi ch'üan is not a by-product, as it were, of any other art-dance form; it is not derived from ancient Chinese commemorative dance, folk, or classical Chinese theater dance, and does not resemble them in dynamics, rhythm, or structure. T'ai-chi ch'üan is a complete entity, composed to answer the needs to which it is directed. Total in concept, it is a synthesis of form and function. With the elements of structure and movement so consummately composed, it is an art in the deepest sense of the word. Aesthetically, it can be compared to a composition by Bach or a Shakespearean sonnet. However, t'ai-chi ch'üan is not art directed outward to an audience. It is an art-in-action for the doer; the observer, moved by its beauty, can only surmise its content. The *experience* of the form in process of change makes it an art for the self.

My intention in writing this book is to bring to the attention of Western people this ancient masterpiece of health exercise, which, ancient though it is, is supremely suitable in these modern times. I wish to create an informed understanding of what is necessary, theoretically, for a vital life, and also to arouse the interest and willingness of the reader to apply this exercise for his or her own use. As an exercise that demands no physical strength to begin with, it therefore is as good for the weak as for the well, for young and old, men and women. Since the techniques are adjusted to, and develop with, individual capacities, it is practical for any disposition.

I do not approach t'ai-chi ch'üan as a mystery or as something mystical. My basic approach is practical in the sense that as a concretely demonstrable exercise, it can be learned and profitably used by anyone, whatever the personality, interests or however limited the level of experience.

Since the integrated nature of this physical exercise is such that the mind and the emotions are simultaneously involved with the action, the doer is enveloped by and made conscious of the physical, emotional, and mental centers from the very beginning of study, even without ever really trying to do so.

More than this, its practicality includes a world of ideas which invigorate the mind, ideas which can be absorbed theoretically even by those who have not participated in the physical practice. This world of ideas includes the aesthetic as well as the scientific, the moral-ethical as well as the utilitarian.

The word "practical" therefore includes: the way the mind functions and the way the emotions affect the physical body, as well as a philosophy of behavior. It is eminently practical to consider our emotional, mental, and physical natures working together as a totality. Movement by movement, step by step, with its organic and intrinsic harmony, it trains both body and mind — to longer life with heightened interest and deeper understanding. The calmness that comes from harmonious physical activity and mental perception and the composure that comes from deep feeling and comprehension are the very heart of this exercise.

T'ai-chi ch'üan can be defined from many points of view: some emphasize content and others, the way of the Method. Awareness of the 'way' will reveal its content; recognition or appreciation of its content will make the 'way' more comprehensible.

Since the exercise includes all aspects simultaneously — method and material, action and thought, technique and content — I offer several succinct characterizations of t'ai-chi ch'üan.

- It is an integrated exercise-art, a Chinese system of activating the body for physical, emotional and mental well-being, as well as for the attainment of higher levels of consciousness.
- It is a method for developing concentration based on the discipline of body-action with mind as the agent or regulator.
- It is designed to develop a stable, integrated personality which state of being contains calmness as well as astuteness (perceptivity, sensitivity).
- It leads to tranquility; with the development of physical stamina and awareness, emotional security blossoms of its own accord.
- It is a mental culture based on structural movements which obey the physiological laws of nature and the law of change, consistently regulating body-forms to be always in complete gravitational balance.
- It exemplifies the harmonious relationship that can take place between mind and body through the organic process of manipulating the total body with unique arrangements meticulously timed and spaced; as a result, inner and outer equilibrium is easily maintained.

This is being practical in the highest sense — to make body and mind function as one in unity. Physical attributes can be mentally conceived; mental attributes can be physically achieved. Flexibility includes agile joints and also quickness of mind. To control unnecessary expenditure of energy is also to be sensitively aware of the state of one's body movements; stable vitality and balanced strength imply calmness and ease and are achieved through the knowledge of how powerful the subtle can be.

Although it takes direct experience from practice for the inner essence of t'ai-chi ch'üan to reveal itself, it is nevertheless possible (and desirable) to perceive intellectually the extent and the intent of the philosophical attitudes of t'ai-chi ch'üan, and also to recognize the concrete values to be derived from it. To appreciate t'ai-chi ch'üan through words will not inhibit the eventual experience. On the contrary, the intellectual appreciation will enhance the experience as one advances step by step, day by day, in actualizing the concepts and in bringing them to life.

Philosophical understanding, enlightened by the word, suits the action in this most tangible of philosophies. Developing oneself through reflective thought and purposeful ideas, concrete and abstract, plus the *doing*—the body activity—will truly make t'ai-chi ch'üan comprehensible as a profound experience. As a *from-the-mind* exercise, meaning the mind as the source (instigator) for body activity, t'ai-chi ch'üan can be understood partially by the *mind* of the reader.

The wonderful thing about writing a book on this subject is that its principles are constantly under one's fingers, for immediate use. When one is blooming and content, to practice it gives greater growth and awareness. When, working restlessly, impatiently, one has come to an impasse, then to do the exercise as revivifying. It settles the mind, quiets the spirit, smoothes out the emotions. With refreshed mind and unagitated heart, one can take on problems again, as has been the experience of many students in diverse fields of work.

The deep interest and enthusiasm that t'ai-chi ch'üan has aroused in those who practice it and those who have seen it have contributed to my desire to make it available for those who have no teacher. This book is a preparation for those who will study with someone eventually; it is best "that beginners be guided by oral teaching, but nevertheless, if you direct yourself with diligence, skill will take care of itself" (as stated in *T'ai-Chi Ch'uan Ching*, Classic of the Ming Dynasty; see Chapter 5 below). For those who are studying or have studied t'ai-chi ch'üan, this book can be a permanent record for more profound self-study. ". . .In teaching others everything depends on consistency, for it is only through repetition that the pupil makes the material his own." (*I-Ching*, Book of Changes)

In rendering the entire exercise precisely, I have included innumerable details that are not noted in Chinese versions, because there they are taken for granted. We in the West, with no background for these techniques, require more specific, minute, exacting explanations. I have, so to speak, put the microscope on the action, without reinterpreting or changing it. Certain repetitions are unavoidable to open up new perspectives and perceptions.

At this point I must mention that I have omitted certain features not imperative for the Western beginning student. Those are other techniques and skills that the study of this exercise can lead to such as the Art of Self-Defense and Joint Hand Operations. I also do not enlarge upon a very important subject, that of *Ch'i*, variously interpreted as breath, spirit, air or as the nervous system in the latest books. The doctrine of *Ch'i* is an important element that enters into art, aesthetics, science, and philosophy. *Ch'i* is a *vital* force differentiated from *life* force; it is the rhythm of nature, the creative principle that makes life. It is circulation and the circular movement of breath within one, an aspect that t'ai-chi ch'üan is greatly concerned with at an advanced stage of development—*Ch'i* is "an urge or energy, compounded of spirit and in a mysterious way the physical breath". (E. Herbert in *Taoist Notebook*)

The Chinese people are prepared philosophically and psychologically for the theory and practice of t'ai-chi ch'üan. An accepted method of movement, it is available everywhere; they have only to reach out for it, to walk to the park (literally), and it can be learned. The degree to which we in the West are *not* prepared for it has governed the choice of the material in this book. In doing so I have kept in mind that an old Chinese idea of proven value is being presented in a new western environment.

The principles, qualities, and features inherent in the nature of this exercise are faithfully given, as taught to me by Grandmaster Ma Yüeh-Liang. However, I have expatiated upon them in order to clarify and emphasize their content. I have consciously included personal aesthetic and psychological interpretations, which have inevitably come from my advanced experience with this exercise, and which are the result of my inquiring into related fields.

## Historical Background: A Consistent Heritage

A great creator of a great work may be considered to represent the culmination of the spirit of his age. In crediting the philosopher Chang San-Feng of the Sung Dynasty (circa eleventh century) with being the father of t'ai-chi ch'üan, this indeed may be true. Chang San-Feng reflected in his work the intellectual (Confucian) and the spiritual-mystical (Taoist) speculations of his time. He changed and expanded the various exercise systems, creating new forms and techniques, and integrating structure with a style which evolved from his deep experiences and philosophical observations.

The principles that are the very heart of t'ai-chi ch'üan were derived from the theories and practices of the different ancient Chinese philosophic schools concerned with the development of man's intrinsic and potential powers. Though intriguing subtleties as to man's ultimate destiny may have divided one school from another, all seem to have agreed that is necessary to achieve both heart-calm (tranquility) and physical health, in order to become a stable, harmonious, realized person. Over the centuries since 2000 B.C.E., philosophers and physicians, alchemists and athletes, have offered their various theories and techniques on: (1) how to combat illnesses of mind and body; (2) how to create the skill of maintaining one's health; (3) how to increase one's power and potentialities; (4) and, after restoring the body to its proper harmony, how to open the way to the understanding of qualities hidden deep within the nature of man—to make him an instrument of his own will.

Even from the earliest times in China, a distinction was made among various forms and functions of designed body-action: (1) those created for commemorative and ritual purposes; (2) those intended to stimulate and influence the minds and hearts of the audience; (3) those used to stimulate and direct the feelings, body, and the mind of the doer himself. These last were termed medical or health gymnastic movement. Along with arithmetic, music, writing and dance for ceremony, the dance for health was included in the liberal arts.

Whatever expressive form the "act of moving" had taken—whether it was the ancient ritual where the priests and shamans danced to honor the "spirits", or whether, as in communal dance, it was to express joy because of a fine harvest—each unmistakably contributed to the idea that body-movement, rhythmically arranged and styled according to physiological and emotional principles, can correct body ills and perpetuate the life force in man.

In ancient China, during Emperor Yü's time (circa 2205 B.C.E.) stagnant waters from a devastating flood had infested the land. Suspecting that the contamination had resulted from the unmoving waters, the Emperor ordered that a series of exercises, called the Great Dances, be done regularly by all the people. The reasoning was simple and obvious: if inactive waters became diseased, the same could be true of inactive bodies. By doing exercises to stimulate the circulation of the blood, the body would be constantly refreshed, making it impervious to disease. Emperor Yü doubtless was putting into practice theories on circulation inherited from his ancestors who believed that "the blood current flows continuously in a circle and never stops. . .it flows like the current of a river...the heart regulates all the blood of the body...unceasing circle movement which is life—circulation is the vital current." These concepts, from the year 2600 B.C.E. (according to the Classic of Medicine, *Nei Ching*, compiled in the third century B.C.E.) accepted in our modern world form the scientific basis of the physical aspect of t'ai-chi ch'uan.

These ancient dances dictated by Yü thus appear to have evolved from movements invented for the cure of diseases a thousand years earlier. Though healing with herbs and plants is known to have been practiced even prior to 3000 B.C.E., exercise persisted as an essential, necessary part of curative and preventative medicine. Nearly every medical prescription had its related exercise, but there were many more exercises than medical recipes.

"Prevention is the best cure" was known in ancient China and may have been the inspiration for the many self-health-exercise systems, since it was said: "Medicine is useful only in *curing* disease."

It was believed that "worry and anxiety cause sickness because they hinder breathing, thus interfering with blood circulation". Thus to do exercises for the physical body only was not enough to insure health. "If the mind is peaceful every joint will feel good. . .and joy quickens the circulation" reflect the belief that body and mind inextricably affect each other.

Confucius said that the *virtuous* live long. The definition of being virtuous, in this case, included having a peaceful heart, a good body, and an active mind. With such balanced personality, "one's behavior could not possibly be improper."

Many streams of philosophic thought contributed to the development of body and mind in harmony, whether it was for "immortality," for long life, or for a better life. All schools included systematic regimes to neutralize the body, by making it so healthy that it would not disturb the mind's growth. "Fatigue your body and you exhaust your mind" was a maxim that clearly compressed this idea of body-mind relationship, as did "clear the intellect and prolong life." The early Taoists (fifth century B.C.E.), withdrawing from active society, stressed the observation of nature and natural phenomena as an essential part of their philosophy. This interest led them, among other things, to the study of man's movements in relation to the way man functions physically, emotionally, intellectually and spiritually. Over the many centuries, their followers evolved patterns, postures, rhythmic movements and breathing exercises that were intended "to develop a clear intellect, ensure good health, and cure complaints."

Complaints, such as indigestion, asthma, sciatica, tuberculosis, heart ailments, eye and skin diseases (to mention but a few of the "hundred illnesses") could be relieved, so it was claimed, by specialized postures and exercises done systematically. Remedies for mental and emotional disturbances were given equal consideration. Bad or disquieting dreams, grief, languor, "ills of the heart", seemingly baseless fears, indolence, "liking savoury things," and insanity were carefully prescribed for. Man's mental, physical and emotional health were always considered together, as an entity.

In the early centuries B.C.E., the techniques to develop the skill in maintaining health and the power to improve it were of immense importance. Gymnastic exercise, or medical movement, besides being a remedy for disease, was made a branch of education for the healthy person as well. "As a means to long life," said Chuang Tzu, philosopher of the Taoist (fourth century B.C.E.) school, "pass some time like a dormant bear." "Imitate the flappings of a duck, the ape's dance, the owl's fixed stare, the tiger's crouch, the pawings of a bear," said others in this time (from a Taoist notebook by Edward Herbert). There was no school of thought, alchemy or medicine which did not include physical culture as a basic necessity for health and spirituality.

The term applied to "medical" exercises is *Kung-Fu*, meaning "work-man" or "work-done", implying that the man himself does the remedial work for himself. Stimulation imposed upon him from the outside by doctors or masseurs was considered by some to be a "degraded form of body training." The conscious control which he exerts upon himself is the most advantageous method for "self-improvement." It was believed that "the mechanism is assisted by placing the body in many different attitudes and postures, in assorted positions of all kinds". Such combinations produce healthful physiological changes, to be used to treat diseases, and by isolation and nonmovement of one part in relation to another moving part, profound improvements would result.

The study of what movements to combine, what to separate, what particular articulations are necessary, resulted in an enormous number of arrangements, permutations, and combinations. To these were added a system of breathing and various positions of lying, standing, sitting, moving (leaps, runs, walks, etc.), combining the elements of activity and passivity. Kung-Fu accomplishes the cure of infirmities, restores harmony in the body, and therefore man, when not disturbed by irregularities, "is freed from the servitude of the senses." The roots of t'ai-chi ch'üan are embedded in the rich soil of such thought.

In the third century of this era, Hua T'o, a surgeon who had experimented with anesthetics, stressed the physical and emotional values of exercise. In a lecture to one of his disciples (as recorded in the *History of Chinese Medicine* by Drs. K. C. Wong and Wu Lien-Teh), Hua T'o said, "The body needs exercise, only it must not be done to the point of exhaustion. . . .It promotes free circulation of the blood and prevents sickness. The used doorstep never rots, so the body. That is why the ancients practiced the bear's neck. . . .and moving the joints to prevent old age. I have a system of exercise called the frolics of the five animals. . .the tiger, deer, bear, monkey, and bird. It removes disease, strengthens the legs, and ensures health. If one *feels out of sorts*, just practice one of these frolics. . ." "To promote sweating and to give feeling of lightness," jumping, twisting, swaying, crawling, swinging contractions and extensions were prescribed, and it was recommended that they be done regularly. Later systems, such as t'ai-chi ch'üan, were guided by the principle that exercise which is truly health-promoting must never exhaust or fatigue, but, on the contrary, should build up a greater energy and produce a feeling of contentment.

Between the second and the tenth centuries C.E., innumerable gymnastic systems evolved, each created for specific purposes. Especially important were the technical contributions made by the many "religious" sects, each in its own secret society. Inasmuch as there had been no medical or philosophical systems that did not include physical culture, these sects, too, made the training of the body an indispensable requirement for becoming a sage and for health and longevity. In the philosophy of Lao-Tzu (sixth century B.C.E.) are admonitions for using one's superior abilities for the common good of society. Different secret groups, at various periods in China's long history, put their physical skills to practical use, "to improve the world and better the lives of the people." An instance of this is the activity of the Yellow Turbans, a sect that aided the final fall of the decaying Han Dynasty at the end of the second century C.E.. They fought unarmed because no "common people" were allowed to carry weapons at this time. Fighting in "unarmed combat" required special techniques and rigorous training, which necessitated the development of new forms and styles. What is important to stress as being pertinent to t'ai-chi ch'üan is the fact that with these physical disciplines, the principle that mind and body together produce perfect prowess was never forgotten.

Inevitably, by the fourth century of the Common Era, following a thousand years of intensive attention to physical-mental health, many separate styles matured, each proclaiming its own physiological and philosophical point of view. A fourth century C.E. boxer wrote a "Canon for Developing the Sinews." Another wrote a treatise on "Deep Breathing As It Relates to Movement." "Lessons for Tensing Movements" became very popular. Exercises in slow and fast tempos were experimented with. Posture-attitudes, allied to philosophy, became an important part of various cults. All were designed for the improvement of health—physical, mental and spiritual.

None of these forms was associated with the arts, because the different objectives of dance and gymnastic were never lost sight of or confused. Nevertheless these exercises had a structural form and a designed composition which we have come to associate with art, and which contribute vitally to the final objective of experiencing an emotional satisfaction and a sense of equilibrium.

In the sixth century, when Buddhist influences, merging with Taoist thought, impregnated the art of painting and the philosophy of ideas and behavior, an Indian monk (called Ta Mo in China) settled down in China at the Shao Lin Monastery. It appears that at this particular period, in contrast to the preceding centuries, and in this particular retreat, the monks were not aware of the necessity of having physical health in order to attain mystical experience. Ta Mo instituted a series of systematic exercises to revivify the enfeebled and emaciated monks, mentally and physically. His Eighteen Form Lohan Exercise, he said, "would transform the body into a strong abode, to provide the soul with a dwelling place." Named for the monastery, his Shao Lin style represents the technique of the "outer-extrinsic" school of exercise (*Wai Chia*). In this "outer" type, muscular action is intense and visible, dynamics are strong and unvaried, energy is external and forcibly produced. Although primarily used for self-defense purposes and for wrestling, it is also practiced today as a personal exercise, since this style too includes the aim of becoming tranquil, as well as being strong.

Another point of view as to what "way of movement" could best prolong life and rejuvenate it was being formulated at this time. Called the soft "inner-intrinsic" school (*Nei Chia*), this technique gave rise to various styles of t'ai-chi ch'üan that are in practice today.

It is known that during the T'ang Dynasty (circa C.E. 750) several different kinds of Kung-Fu (not yet called Ch'üan) were in practice. A long-bearded philosopher, Hsü Hsuan-P'ing (a wood cutter by trade) performed a "Long Kung-Fu," in which the patterns were continuously connected. The ingredients of *length* and *continuity* added a new element to the philosophy of mental discipline and to the science of increasing physical endurance. Of the thirty-seven Forms comprising his Long Kung-Fu, Hand Strums the Lute, Single Whip, Seven Stars, Jade Girl, High-Pat the Horse, Phoenix (Stork or Crane in today's version) Flaps Its Wings, are Forms that are in t'ai-chi ch'üan today. During this period several other Kung-Fu having this character of "continuity" were being practiced: "Heavenly-Inborn," "Nine Small Heavens" and "Acquired Kung-Fu." These early forms were the seeds from which the 108 Forms of t'ai-chi ch'üan flowered.

By the Sung Dynasty (after C.E. 1000), the concept of "the inner-intrinsic" school (*Nei Chia*) was firmly established. This system emphasized "soft" movement as being the best technique for loosening the joints, circulating the blood, and building up a reserve of energy, with the philosophy that the mind must be in control of action, and that through this method, since "man was capable of wonders," he could fulfill himself as a superior, "realized" human being. Among the many philosophers engaged in the pursuit of such fulfillment, and who consistently practiced various ch'üan, was Chang San-Feng, who was over ninety when he died.

He was sixty-seven years old, when, after thirty-five years of study, he settled down at the Wu Tang Monastery for nine years. During this time he created his version of ch'üan, and his "way" was completed. Linking older Forms, changing and augmenting them, he evolved a unified system utilizing the principle of the t'ai-chi, which, when in action, separates into yin and yang. They say that he was inspired by the play of the contrasting movements of the bird and the serpent—the firm and the yielding. Alternating yin and yang in continuous succession, and with the principle of "controlling the active by means of the quiet," he created his ch'üan from the point of view of philosophy and physiology, psychology, geometry and the law of dynamics. Opposed to hardness, he stressed elasticity, and made a distinction between nature giving strength (physical) and man giving strength (will-power).

His inner-intrinsic school of exercise (*Nei Chia*) is known as the Wu Tang school from the monastery where it was, so to speak, synthesized. This vital system is said to embrace the most permanent, profound, and scientific aspects of its predecessors. Its scope was extended to include a technique for heightening perception and increasing the ability to concentrate and co-ordinate, of activating the mind, and of producing a harmonious equilibrium of thought and action for the attainment of tranquility. The concept of *t'ai-chi ch'üan* dates from Chang San-Feng's time.

The various styles came into being during the ensuing centuries. The Wu Style is a variation of the original Yang style and was created by Wu Chuan Yü (1834-1902). The other styles also take their names from their originators. Mr. Ma Yüeh-Liang (my teacher of the Wu style) believes that "some creations are improvements of previous inventions and are better than the former because the new ones have been able to eliminate mistakes and have had more time to perfect themselves." The Wu Style in the book to follow is a perfection of centuries of development, and it preserves the classic length, detail and subtlety.

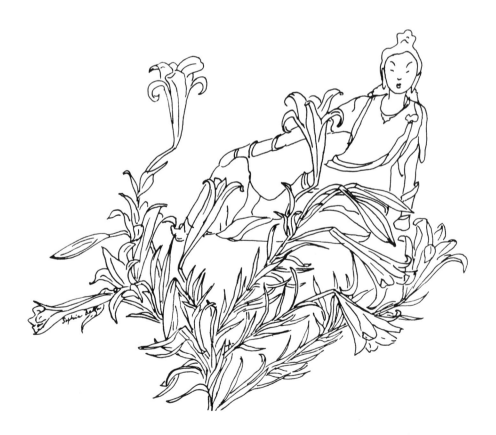

# Part One:

*The Way Of T'ai-Chi Ch'üan*

T'ai chi ch'üan is a form of ch'üan. What is ch'üan? Ch'üan means fist; metaphorically, action. The word connotes power and control over one's own actions: the epitome of organized movement, the ultimate in protection of the self. To be expert in ch'uan is to have immunity—immunity from destructive external forces and from poor health. It is also to have the power to control the self. The uses of this power and the ends toward which it is to be directed depend entirely upon the inclinations and interests of the individual; these may range from the purely physical to the philosophic or spiritual.

To us in the West, a fist provocatively denotes aggressive attack. In ancient Chinese thought, a fisted hand, on the contrary, meant concentration, isolation, and containment, as depicted in wood blocks showing figures in various exercising positions (Kung-Fu) with fisted hands. We can assume that ch'üan implies the active as controlled by the inactive—the active being form or matter and the inactive being spirit or mind.

As a synonym for exercise, with deep implications as to its usefulness, ch'üan is a technique of organized harmonious forms. Its essence is continuity of action where each movement evolves from and grows out of what it is joined to, motivating and spurring on the subsequent movement. The correspondence between the parts of the body is essential to structure, idea, and feeling. "One single movement suffices to affect other movements." "No isolated rest without eventually enveloping the whole." "Just as in the turning flow of a stream, so the positions are determined by the spaces between."

Symbolically, ch'üan is mental and physical co-ordination. If the body is in fine health, then the mind can function skillfully and adroitly. The body is the form, and the mind, which is the spirit, is actually the moving force. Mental "motion" is present with every physical action. T'ai-chi ch'üan is "controlled by the mind" exercise (*Ting Tou Yuan*).

What is T'ai-chi? T'ai-chi is the concept that all of life is composed of, and has been set in motion by, the constant interplay of two vital energies: yin, the passive, and yang, the active principle. "T'ai-chi is the mother of yin and yang (everything female and male)," which has given rise to everything under the sun.

No part has a life of its own, but each exists in complementary interaction with the other. "Yin and Yang mutually help each other." "T'ai-chi is the root of motion (yang) which has division, and of stillness (yin) which has union." T'ai-chi *is* this duality in harmonious relationship.

The symbol for the T'ai-chi is a circle divided into two curved shapes of equal size, one being yin, the shadowed right part, the other yang, the light part. A touch of yin in yang and of yang in yin is indicated by the

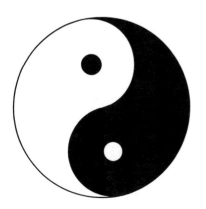

small spot or dot of the opposite color in each area, showing the flexible and sympathetic character of each to the other. The line between them has the movement of a wave. The fall and rise of the wave-line is also yin and yang; this flowing is restrained and contained by the evenness of the circumference. All of this movement represents the continuity of the life force, which is *movement*.

Yin as the receptive, feminine, and yang as the creative, masculine, complement each other. Though opposite, they are not in opposition or antagonistic. Though different, they supplement each other. In the continuous movement between them, without beginning and without end, when yang reaches its final moment, then yin is created and starts. The interplay of these two fundamental and vital elements implies "perpetual motion." Together, in T'ai-chi, where their relationship is perfect, they constitute equilibrium and harmony.

T'ai-chi holds in balance what is separated. A few examples of the opposites (placing the yang before the yin) as experienced in the exercise of t'ai-chi ch'üan, are movement-stillness, motion-rest, tangible-intangible, straight-curved, expansion-contraction, inhalation-exhalation, outside-inside, solid-empty (void), light-dark, firm-soft, open-closed, right-left, forward-backward, float-settle, and rise-sink. There is nothing without its opposite; there is nothing that does not change (move) in order to be permanent (to live)—which in itself is a yin-yang statement.

We in the West are apt to overexert ourselves in exercise and sports, believing that a hard and tense movement indicates strength and control, and that power comes from the ability to expend energy violently. The spirit of t'ai-chi ch'üan is the antithesis of such a point of view. With the technique of t'ai-chi ch'üan, true energy can be controlled, strength balanced, and vitality increased, by using the body in such a way as *not* to strain the muscles, not to overactivate the heart, *not* to exert oneself excessively. It is in the philosophy of t'ai-chi ch'üan that in order to prolong the life of the body, to stabilize the life of the emotions, and to intensify the life of the mind, conscious co-operation of the mind with activity is a deep necessity. For certainly peace of mind cannot be attained without the use of the mind. The consideration of man's total health as an inseparable unity is evident in every moment of this long, slow exercise.

## Benefits

The practice of t'ai-chi ch'üan is a way to develop both body and mind to such a degree that "one can retard old age and make spring eternal." At the same time it strengthens and revitalizes the body, it helps "the cultivation of a calm heart," and enables the mind to function with more awareness, clarity and concentration.

In *The Body*, Anthony Smith writes that in strenuous exercise the muscles need more and in fact get more of the body's blood distribution *but* at the expense of the other organs: kidneys, skin, digestive system and stomach. As one example, the abdomen, which ordinarily receives 24% gets only *one*% during supreme exertion.

T'ai-chi ch'üan as an instrinsic exercise increases the blood circulation and activity of the glands, nourishes muscles, facilitates joint action and stimulates the nervous system, all without increasing the activity of the heart or breathing rhythm. The technique, circular in nature, soft, slow, and continuous, and above all subscribing to the principles of yin and yang, affects the entire system in a superior way, involving every organ as well as the surface skin. T'ai-chi ch'üan properly harmonizes the circulation of the various vital currents and, so to speak, unties the knots or pressures blocking the process of assimilation.

As a healing art, t'ai-chi ch'üan serves as a remedy for high blood pressure, anemia, joint diseases and gastric disturbances, and has been used as a cure for tuberculosis.

T'ai-chi ch'üan aims also at "the cultivation of temperament". The balance of movements and the way of using slowness, lightness, and calmness relax nervous temperaments, give one an easy pace and "therefore a good disposition," and "rid one of arrogance and conceit." Because every movement is anticipated by the mind, patience and control of temper develop without effort; a consistent equilibrium between the heart and mind is established.

We know very well that dynamic interest is beneficial to one's nervous system, and that a happy spirit and an enthusiastic frame of mind can affect health favorably. And being in a state of good health can exhilarate one's spirits. With a good nervous system one's whole being becomes more perceptive, alert, and receptive.

The benefits of t'ai-chi ch'üan are intellectual and psychological, too. One can more easily adjust oneself to meet the various and continuously changing stimuli of one's environment with steady equanimity.

With an increase of intrinsic energy, one's interest is heightened. Because the techniques involve change and nuance, awareness and mental alertness, one becomes more sensitive and capable of greater understanding. The mind is concentrated. This basic principle of concentration in which the mind directs the energy and the energy in turn exercises the body, is a key factor in attaining the final objectives: acquiring energy without tenseness, strength without hardness, vitality without nervousness, and especially achieving tranquility. This is not the tranquility of inaction, but the tranquility of the following definition from *I-Ching*, Book of Changes:

> Tranquility is a kind of vigilant attention. It is when tranquility is perfect that the human faculties display all their resources, because then they are enlightened by reason and sustained by knowledge.

This definition sums up the Chinese point of view, essential in the study of t'ai-chi ch'üan.

The technique of t'ai-chi ch'üan is based on a way of movement that significantly involves the Forms, with a styled method of making the pattern evolve from the movement, and the movement from the Forms.

The structures are so varied as to put into play every part of the body from the smallest joint to the largest muscle. Harmoniously designed and masterfully patterned, they are done with flowing continuity. Slowness, evenness, clarity, balance and calmness are the five basic qualities of the composite technique. The perfect weaving of the dynamics of movement and form promotes fine circulation, and, above all, quiets the mind and regulates the emotions.

In the very first place, it is the "softness" of this style of exercise which develops energy—by never allowing one to expend oneself in a gesture of finality. This softness contrasts with the hard or energetic force that does *not* permit such reserve of action. Natural body behavior with a style of moving in fluid and continuous motion "like the movement of a never-ending river" eliminates any possiblity of becoming rigid or hard.

The great play of dynamics contained in t'ai-chi ch'üan is so utilized that no one part of the body can be overstrained. Because of the constant alternating interplay of action, one's whole system feels neither a beginning nor an end of movement, from which a state of emotional equilibrium is created.

The immense variety of patterns keeps one mentally stimulated as the techniques develop from Form to Form. The mind cannot be anywhere *but* on the action since the variations and repetitions demand total attention. Because the structure does not evolve correctly without this mind participation, control of the consciousness develops inevitably. Concentration is a natural result of such technique and form.

Moving in slow time prevents the body from becoming tense or hard and makes muscles resilient and pliable. Strength cannot be wasted or falsely propelled, because slow movement requires attentive control.

The entire system is warmed up gradually as the action accumulates. Patterns and movements, in subtle succession, activate different parts of the body, and never at any time repeat themselves in overconcentrated units. This enables the body to do more without making the heart beat faster to keep up with the body changes.

Breathing is natural—light or deep depending on the structure and the positions of the Forms themselves. However, beginners must not concern themselves with the breathing process. This aspect is developed in the advanced study of t'ai-chi ch'üan.

The fundamentally slow and unvarying basic tempo contributes to the ability to sustain conscious control and aids in building up reserves of energy. With the flowing alternation of light and strong dynamics of void and solid forms, energy circulates freely to all parts of the body.

The movement requires that motion be outwardly unvarying and in continuous flow. Ability to maintain a consistently slow tempo and an even quality over a long period of time is an indication, not only that the body has acquired strength and control, but also that the mind is in harmony with the action.

Personal moods and distracting emotions evaporate as one is taken out of oneself by attention to motions and forms that are completely objective and impersonal. In this way, one understands oneself without subjective interference.

In terms of pure movement, the patterns are so constructed that the strong alternates with the light, the active with the quiescent, the weighted with the empty, the solid with the void, expansion with contraction—the relationships being as flexible and continuous as the form of the wave line within the t'ai-chi.

Within a design or movement structure, one part of the body may be still while another part is active; one hand in a yin position and the other yang. All the weight, with controlled force, may be held on one side, while the other is light and receptive, an opposite relationship taking place in the following sequence, with differently designed arrangements. No muscle, joint, limb, no part of the body is ever overtaxed or underactivated. Both excess and deficiency are avoided, since each is contrary to the philosophy of t'ai-chi ch'üan.

## Structure (Yin-Yang)

Not only are the elements of yin-yang apparent in the movement and design from pattern to pattern, no matter how minute, but they are contained also in the structure of the Forms, which are composites of many designs.

In going from one design to another, the connecting line is so deliberately controlled that it is as smooth, as unvarying, as continuous as a circle. Though the Form is constantly changing from yin to yang, the external appearance never shows that there are changes in the dynamics of muscular tension. In this "soft-intrinsic" exercise, the outer appearance is soft, and the inner force is firm, whereas in "hard-intrinsic" exercise, the dynamics, always intense, are never varied.

Yin-yang appears in the exerciser's attitude as well. The strength used to manipulate the body is not registered on the face; the spirit is calm, and, therefore, the face is quiet and the look is effortless. This is *not* deception. It is exactly how one feels, because the intrinsic nature of this technique gives the doer the feeling of containment while being active.

Because the inner control that the action demands is not apparent to the observer, the action seems weightless, airy, easy, thoughtless, and soft without energy. But the weightlessness actually is of such substance that "motion is like refined steel." What seems to be easy is "as controlled as a hawk trying to catch a rabbit." It is "as thoughtless as a cat waiting to catch a mouse" where attention and concentration are completely centered. The softness has "the reserve of energy of a bow about to be snapped." Inside one is firm, stable, controlled, and at the same time the appearance is of repose and effortlessness. This is yin-yang in its relation to the outside world.

## Harmony of Body and Mind

The way of movement is, in a deeper sense, related to the "movement of the mind". The mind must direct the body movement; the mind wills and the body behaves. The alertness and concentration needed to do this are developed as the Forms are being mastered.

One of the great advantages of t'ai-chi ch'üan is that one can never be automatic when doing it. The body and personality are one in action. The benefit of this is perhaps obvious, since t'ai-chi ch'üan has, as one of its goals, the development of awareness and consciousness, quickened reflexes, and an alert mind.

The mind can be directed to control the body at a fraction of a moment's notice. The action is so designed that the logical follow-through is upset if the mind absents itself. The astutely composed themes and the artful arrangements of detailed designs bring the attention back from its undirected wanderings, forcing one to be doubly attentive. This is truly an exercise *with* the mind, training it to function consistently and harmoniously with the will.

To omit any of the repeated Forms, in addition to weakening the mental concept of t'ai-chi ch'üan, will ruin its structure, which has philosophical and artistic meaning. The composition of the structure is explicit as to floor pattern, space, and design.

The structure arouses a sense of aesthetic appreciation, a satisfaction that comes from the balanced harmony of a perfectly arranged work of art. The repeated Forms, spaced with psychological insight, give mental rest and physical ease, because at certain points in the development of the exercise, it is necessary *not* to have a new problem. The exercise ends exactly in the footprints where it started. The significance of t'ai-chi ch'üan's ending and starting as it does is that it gives to the performer a sense of the whole, which, though completed, can inevitably resume its motion.

The co-ordination aspect of movement within movement and design within design demands complete attention. The subtle regulation of the timing of each small part within the whole *is* co-ordination. The mind moves from form, to style, to tempo, to co-ordination, to plasticity, to dynamics, to "feeling," and yet seems to acknowledge all at the same time. Concentrated by this variety, mind, attention, and awareness are one.

The mental habit of concentration acquired from these techniques is easily carried over to other subjects, which is another way of saying that when mind and body are in harmony, anything that must be done, can be done with the complete co-operation of mind, will, and feeling. The techniques of t'ai-chi ch'üan give thought to action and action to thought with the mind in control. The profound and minutely brilliant detail in the exercise patterns prods, coaxes , and leads one into the clear path of heightened awareness. Awareness overcomes restlessness. The act of consciously focusing attention can, almost instantly, make one calm, when in action or at rest.

## Two Intrinsic Principles: Softness and Circular Movement

*Softness.* This "inner" or soft school of movement can easily be recognized by the fact that there is *no* visible exertion in the execution of the movements. The action and the person appear to be completely relaxed because the activity is hidden inside, below the surface. The continuous flow of movement into movement, without straining, also contributes to this outer "soft" appearance. Actually, all the movements are done with controlled inner force. It is not the extent to which movement can go that matters; rather it is the quality in reserve that determines its softness, which means "intrinsic-stored up-within." With this soft technique the body can be held loosely and circulation is therefore unrestricted. This helps store up intrinsic energy and makes an elasticity which is "inside and yet is rich in power of resilience."

With continuity and slowness as component parts of softness, calmness and lightness are the inevitable results. No matter what the movements — pushing, pressing, lifting, stretching, leg-lifts, or deep charges — because of this development of soft elasticity, the breath never comes quickly, nor is the heart beat accelerated. Flexibility and vigor are developed without forced effort.

*Circular Movement.* T'ai-chi ch'üan is often referred to as the circular exercise because all patterns and designs (with the obvious necessary exception) are composed of circles, curves, arcs, parabolas, and spirals of all sizes, which go in many directions — horizontal, vertical, or slanted. They may move in opposition or concurrently, and in various tempi. (See pages 168-173).

This technique is not arbitrary or just abstractly decorative. The act of weaving and interrelating the patterns in a circular way evokes calmness and creates energy. By limiting the extent of the action, circular motion helps to reserve energy. It prevents one from overexpending oneself, since the dynamics of physical tension can be controlled when moving in the line of a curve. The sustained ability to move continuously in a curve increases strength and endurance.

Circular motion, where there appears to be no ending to the gestures and no corners to the designs, creates evenness which is an important factor in relaxing the tenseness of body and mind. A circle of movement produces a sense of detachment, containment, and emotional security.

All the diverse circular units in the exercise are balanced by evenly paced action and by the control of the center of gravity. This combination resembles the symbol for T'ai-chi, in which the outer circle equilibrates the movement within it. By maintaining the circular smoothness in action, an outer passivity is attained. Simultaneously, to "balance the opposites," with the activity of the movements, an inner stillness is created.

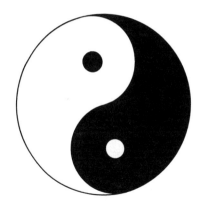

From doing t'ai-chi ch'üan one gets the feeling of perpetual motion. The circle and all its varying forms hold the movements together in a unity of technique and mood. The basic tempo remains unchanged and holds together other varying tempi, which are slower, thus integrating form and space. The precisely designed space in which the body moves is regulated by the patterns of the body composition. Although there is continuing motion, the action is so distributed that no *single* part of the body is in continual motion, or is continually at rest. The yin-yang elements, alternating with regularity, give an impetus to the motion. Here, too, the dynamics of lightness and force, moving from one part of the body to another, keep the action continuous and perpetual.

The body in action is a small universe of multiple movements and synchronized Forms, moving on itself and in space, duplicating, as it were, the composite rotation of the planets, where each, turning in its own rhythm, is in perfect co-ordination with the others in orbit.

### Five Essential Qualities

Slowness, lightness, clarity, balance, and calmness are each the cause and effect of the other. The inner essence and the outer style, the means and the end, are harmoniously one. Through their fluent interplay, the form and spirit of t'ai-chi ch'üan are crystallized.

*Slowness (Man).* It is absolutely essential to move slowly, as slowly as the tempo set for the duration of the entire exercise, which for the beginner is twenty minutes, Even though, as a beginner, you will not be able to sustain an even tempo, you must nevertheless execute the action slowly. This slowness is so basically natural that you cannot but find the right tempo when you start, because the design, from the very first movement, leads you into the proper tempo, provided, of course, that you *think* in terms of moving slowly. Note that no mention has been made of music accompaniment, because no outside stimulus is necessary for this intrinsic exercise. You yourself are in control; you *are* the tempo, the rhythm, the form, and the spirit. As one masters the exercise, the tempo can be slowed down and the total time increased to twenty-five or thirty minutes. When expert, you can, with unerring assurance, prolong the time as you wish, without losing the synchronization of time, space, and form.

There are many reasons for moving with slowness. Slowness aids in the process of developing awareness. You have more time to observe what you are doing, since you are doing half as much in twice the time. Patience and poise come with sustaining slow, physical control.

To be able to move slowly with conscious control dispels ill temper and irritability. When one is nervous, gestures are irregularly fast and staccato. Slow motion soothes the nerves. "To exercise slowly is to be light; to be light is to be calm." With slowness you can savor the movement. Aesthetically, you can appreciate the most delicate turn of the wrist as well as the intangible detail of a large design. You are sensitized to the dynamics of change, to intricacies of pattern, to the weaving of space. You can experience the moment of synchronized stillness and the dovetailing process of movement.

The purely physical power accumulated by means of this slow technique is a reservoir of energy. The ability to fix attention and gather strength develops quick reactions and reflexes. "If one can control slowness, then one can act speedily."

*Lightness (Ch'ing).* This aspect of movement encompasses continuity, softness, regularity, evenness, smoothness and flow. The Chinese image, as it applies to these qualities, relates to a delicate, difficult, patience-demanding occupation—that of getting the silk out of a cocoon intact: "Manipulating outer energy is like pulling silk." To strain and pull is to break the thread. To force motion and to exert falsely put a strain on the system. To overdo is to break the thread, and to underdo is not to get it at all. To have lightness in t'ai-chi ch'üan is to be able to draw out the movement uninterruptedly from beginning to end. This, like the silk, which has tensile strength, will give a sustained vitality with the power of long life.

To have lightness enables one to move flowingly. To move with flow is to be even and continuous; to be continuous is to be endless; to be endless one must move in curves; to move in curves is to be light.

*Clarity (Chieh).* Referring expressly to the mind, this word "clarity" combines the concepts of clean and pure. If the mind can be concentrated on the process of action, it will be cleansed of intruding thoughts. I have taken the liberty of extending the concept of clarity to the physical aspect of the Forms. If the mind is purely directed, then the Forms will be cleanly done. If the Forms are made purely, cleansed of carelessness and inaccuracies, then the mind inevitably has clarity. With the mind alerted, no Form can be vague, nor will the outline of movement be irregular, amorphous, ragged, or inexact. It is with clarity that the mind weaves a wholeness, since it is not merely a matter of doing but also of knowing.

*Balance (Heng).* "Gravity is the root of grace, the mainstay of all speed" (by Lao-tzu, translated by Witter Bynner).

To be well-balanced is to be in full control of both static and mobile equilibrium. Balance applies to the physical and to a state of harmony that is emotional and mental. At every moment in the course of the patterned sequences there is complete and mathematical balance. T'ai-chi ch'üan is unlike any other exercise in that it necessitates having or being in constant balance. When a body is in perfect balance, there is no strain on any part of it.

For balance one must necessarily have (1) physical ability, (2) an understanding of movement sequences, (3) an even flow of movement and control of the inactive, (4) control of the changes from yin to yang and from solid (*Shih*) to empty (*Hsü*), (5) control of movement, from space to form, (6) mental awareness, and (7) a spirit of calmness. All these requirements balance themselves and contribute to the mastery of each part. As gradually and imperceptibly as a root takes hold, as a plant grows, as a stem lengthens, and as flowers mature, so inevitably does balance become serenity. "When a master stands, he is in perfect balance and moves like a carriage wheel."

*Calmness (Ching)*. "Calmness is of decisive importance." You are asked to start with calmness and to make your mind direct the action. In a fraction of a second you can "suspend the torrents of thoughts" by this act of attentiveness. An even-flowing continuity creates calmness. Smooth manipulation of movement sustains this sense of repose; and thus ease of mind grows out of form and technique. With the development of stability, both physical and mental, a state of calmness becomes habitual.

"Action—seek quiet inside," refers to a blending of action and quiet that affects the entire system. Action keeps one from getting too lax, and quietness keeps one from getting too hard.

The everchanging variety of yin and yang, in "peaceful" relationship, gives mental and bodily equilibrium; the structural integration of the Forms, being a work of art as well as a work of science, contains a natural harmony that in itself is calmness.

Without calmness there can be no concentration; without concentration there can be no co-ordination; and without co-ordination there is no harmony.

Slowness, lightness, clarity, balance, and calmness, softness, and circular movement are basic, and are united and interdependent, as are the Forms, between which there are no gaps. Every movement is the instigator of what follows and the result of what has preceded. These qualities are also like harmonious chords in music—simultaneously apparent—where each note responds to the overtones of the others and deeply influences the others' essence. As in the waveline of the T'ai-chi, they move in endless succession; and like its delineating circumference, these elements are fused, without beginning and without end. In t'ai-chi ch'üan, whether one starts with the mind and continues with the body, or starts with the body and continues with the mind, there is always a state of harmony. "Gradual comprehension comes from growing familiarity which leads one to superlative clarity [mastery]". "But unless one pursues this exercise long enough he cannot hope to understand. . .because nothing can be mastered all of a sudden."

I have incorporated technical ideas in this book that have grown out of teaching situations, to give students not only an intellectual awareness of what t'ai-chi ch'üan is, but also to create the understanding with which to experience its essence. We know too well that this process cannot be hurried unnaturally; nevertheless, the way can be illuminated by "quietly studying and analyzing and then one gradually by degrees learns to do the bidding of the mind."

"To go a thousand miles one has to take the first step" is a familiar Chinese saying. Each step, ostensibly, is like the following one, but the added experience that each brings to the next one contributes to endurance, agility, and strength. The act of self-study which by its very nature involves will power, thought, and awareness, is a dynamic step forward. The great variety of Forms and intensely interesting techniques, the subtleties of which unfold with experience, and the sheer beauty of the postures, give delight, even if one has not mastered them, and keep one constantly alert and stimulated. To practice the exercise at any stage of one's development is to be better and to feel better.

As one develops understanding and progresses with the technique, t'ai-chi ch'üan becomes a richer entity, seemingly limitless in what it has to offer. To perform it for its minimum of twenty to twenty-five minutes gives one lasting good health. To perfect it and to live with it as a life-long exercise is to assure oneself of stable health, mental alertness, and equanimity of spirit.

Release yourself from the thought of time pressing in on you. The factor of time enters into the fact of progress. By doing, you begin to know. By knowing, you then begin to do.

The slower the exercise is done, the lighter it looks, but the weightier it feels. Sensations of lightness and strength are simultaneous. Speeding up reveals plasticity; slowing down reveals form. However, for the observer the form seems to be revealed by quick motion and the plasticity by slow movement. Each movement is like a wave in a moving stream; the beginning and the end cannot be seen. To maintain a flowing action, you must have control beneath the surface: the lighter and smoother it looks, the more muscular control it has.

To comprehend is to know mentally; to apprehend is to sense and feel. For t'ai-chi ch'üan you must both know and feel. As a long exercise, it builds up energy gradually. As you grow with it, from two, to five, to ten, and finally to twenty minutes, you are never exhausted, because the development is natural, unstrained, easy, and inevitable.

Note the difference between the slow movement of t'ai-chi ch'üan and the slow motion of a moving picture in which the action is made to move more slowly than is possible in real life, as for example in the artificial slow motion of a diver in space. In t'ai-chi ch'üan, because the body is always in a state of equilibrium and the designs are related to each other in impeccable balance, the movement can be slowed down to an enormous degree, depending on the technique and control of the doer. This is *real* slow motion.

To make legs move in a perfectly flowing way, muscular stamina is needed. To make arms and torso move in a perfectly flowing way, it is not physical strength that is needed; it is concentration and awareness and conscious control.

With concentration there is stillness, in balance there is concentration, and in stillness there is balance. Equilibrium of body, heart, and mind makes one feel "at one with oneself."

"True quiet means keeping still when the time has come to keep still, and going forward when the time has come to go forward. In this way, rest and movement are in agreement. . .with the demands of the time. . .."
*I-Ching*, Book of Changes.

**Principles to be Observed**

1. Always keep in mind: slowness, lightness, clarity, balance, and calmness.
2. Be consistent in tempo.

3. Fix attention on what you are doing at the moment you are doing it.

4. Remember: Approach t'ai-chi ch'üan from the point of view of mind as well as body.

5. Movement is based on the normal, natural way the body functions: keep head straight, waist loose, buttocks in, joints open, and arms easy.

6. If you exercise for strength alone you will lose the spirit; if you exercise for spirit alone you will lose the Form and not achieve the proper spirit.

7. Each movement spurs on the next movement; this is continuous and flowing form.

8. Do not make your steps too small; they must be in correct proportion to your size.

9. You will acquire balance if you distinguish between the Empty and the Solid Steps.

10. Distinguish between the various hand positions: yin, yang, and standing (neutral). Be aware of where the finger tips are directed.

11. Do not exert; do not use all your strength. You should move with springlike tension, capable of great expansion.

12. Distinguish between the active and the inactive parts of your body. One part of your body is in motion all the time, but not the same part.

13. That part of your body which is not in movement must be held firmly, but not rigidly, with conscious control.

14. The upper part of your body—torso and head—must be light. The lower part below the waist controls the weight and solidity. This is the proper body balance—otherwise you would be topheavy, clumsy, and off-balance.

15. Motion follows a circular shape like that of the T'ai-chi symbol, in which there are different degrees of dynamics.

16. Keep the harmonious sequence of feet, knees, legs, waist, hands, and head.

17. Every movement has its counterpart: forward-backward, in-out, up-down, in opposition-together, right-left.

18. Strength comes from the legs not from the forward pressure of the shoulders.

19. Every movement and every small fraction within it is of equal importance. Do not flourish the hand movements; the smaller the movements, the more difficult they are to control in proper tempo.

20. Note the *fast* movements well; these are difficult to do clearly and speedily. Keep in mind the reasons for these patterns: (1) they increase your ability to move from a slow action to a quick one without external

preparation; (2) they increase your ability to recover your basic tempo from a more rapid one without a transition; (3) they center the attention or bring back the attention, if you have been lulled by the slow, flowing movements; (4) and as my teacher Ma Yüeh-Liang laughingly said, "They keep you from getting bored!"

21. Remember: "Attention centers not on things in their state of being but upon their movements in change." *I-Ching*, Book of Changes

**Basic Positions**

It is necessary to become familiar with the basic positions that are part of the technique of t'ai-chi ch'üan. Knowing them well will facilitate the process of learning the Forms as a whole.

Use them as reference but do not utilize them as exercise. Only in the text itself are they done as an exercise together with the movements that precede and follow them. The principle involving the interplay of yin and yang, and of "Empty and Solid," on which the exercise is based, will then not be violated.

1. Posture: Stand straight and be centered (*Chung*), feeling comfortable, easy (*An Shu*), and without tension or strain. To achieve this natural, comfortable position, the head is held straight at "a ninety degree angle to the horizon," so that the top of the head is directed upward. The neck is held tall, lightly and "humbly"—this means without strain or tension, which is arrogant, and without limpness, which is submissive. (Fig. 18)

Shoulders must be low and loose, which frees both neck and back from tenseness. The chest is neither pushed up nor hollowed out. The abdomen must not protrude or be overcontracted.

The spine is straight but not stiff, with buttocks not protruding. If body balance is correct, the hips will be even and level. An overarched spine is a stiff spine, which thrusts hips backward and throws the coccyx out of alignment.

No joint is stiffened or locked. The arms hang in their natural line with loose elbows. (Fig. 1) The legs are straight with knee joints flexible.

The torso should feel light. You should feel firm and supported solidly by the area below the waist and by the legs.

You should feel light "as if suspended by the top of the head," yet so strong that "you could support the world."

2. *Basic Stance* (P'ing Hsing Pu): Place feet parallel and apart, separated by a distance equal to the length of your foot. Your feet are therefore, as it were, set on the sides of a square. "The feet are the earth and the head is heaven." (Fig. 2)

3. *Bent-Knee position*: Take the basic stance with feet parallel and apart. Bend both knees equally; keep back straight as it is lowered by the bending

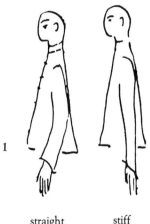

1

straight    stiff

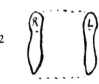

2

Basic Stance

28

of the knees. Feel the active movement at the waist, which must take place when you keep your spine straight and buttocks tucked under. (Fig. 21)

Points of knees are directly over the toes; do *not* let knees pull together.

4.  *Flexed Foot position*, (a) *the Empty Step* (*Hsü Pu*): Take the basic stance with feet parallel and apart. Bend both knees equally. Then move left leg directly forward, raise toes upward, and touch heel to ground lightly. Straighten left knee. Weight is on right leg with its bent knee. There is no weight on left leg. This is the Empty Step, which means that it is empty of any weight. (Observe the feet in Figure 3.) (b) *the Solid Step* (*Shih Pu*) is on that foot which holds the weight. To maintain perfect balance, the transition from Empty to Solid must be carefully controlled.

Each position is made on either foot.

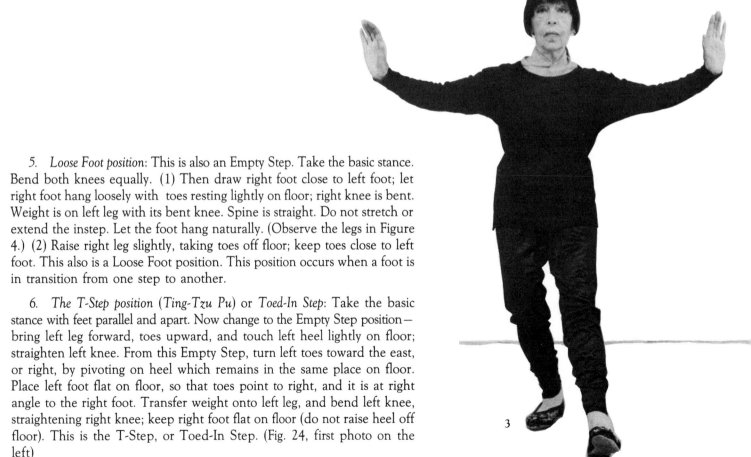

3

5.  *Loose Foot position*: This is also an Empty Step. Take the basic stance. Bend both knees equally. (1) Then draw right foot close to left foot; let right foot hang loosely with toes resting lightly on floor; right knee is bent. Weight is on left leg with its bent knee. Spine is straight. Do not stretch or extend the instep. Let the foot hang naturally. (Observe the legs in Figure 4.) (2) Raise right leg slightly, taking toes off floor; keep toes close to left foot. This also is a Loose Foot position. This position occurs when a foot is in transition from one step to another.

6.  *The T-Step position* (*Ting-Tzu Pu*) or *Toed-In Step*: Take the basic stance with feet parallel and apart. Now change to the Empty Step position— bring left leg forward, toes upward, and touch left heel lightly on floor; straighten left knee. From this Empty Step, turn left toes toward the east, or right, by pivoting on heel which remains in the same place on floor. Place left foot flat on floor, so that toes point to right, and it is at right angle to the right foot. Transfer weight onto left leg, and bend left knee, straightening right knee; keep right foot flat on floor (do not raise heel off floor). This is the T-Step, or Toed-In Step. (Fig. 24, first photo on the left)

This position occurs on either foot.

7.   *Seated position* or *Horse-Riding Step* (*Ch'i Ma Pu*): Separate feet by a space equal to twice the length of your foot. Place toes out at a *slight* angle. Bend both knees equally. Direct knees over toes. Keep back straight and buttocks tucked under. Do not arch the back. Weight is equal on both legs. (Observe legs in Figure 5.)

8.   *The Walking Step position* or *Bow Step* (*Kung Pu*), and the *Walking Step Space*: Take the basic stance with feet parallel and apart facing west (or to the left side of the room). Now bring left leg forward in the Empty Step position (see Figure 3), with left heel touching ground lightly; weight is on right leg with its bent knee. Now transfer weight onto left leg, placing entire foot flat on floor, and bend left knee at the same time. Straighten

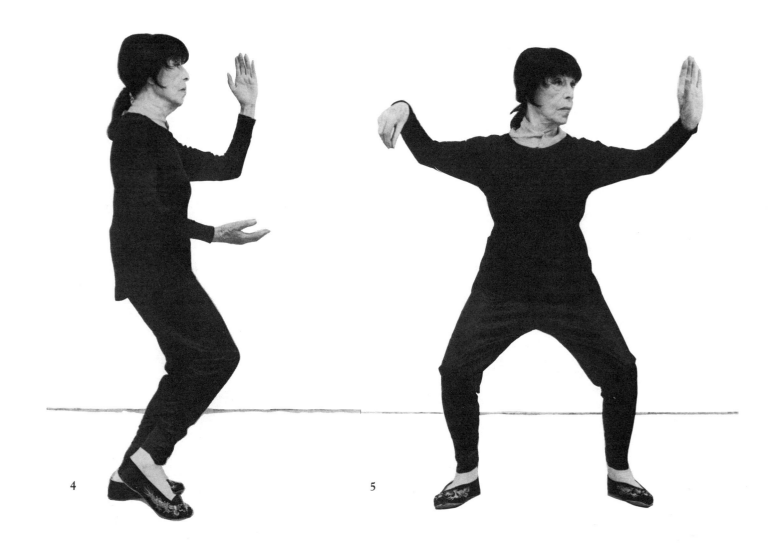

4                                        5

right knee keeping right heel on floor. Torso slants forward on a diagonal with body in a straight line from head to right heel; spine is straight and buttocks remain tucked under. Hips are even, shoulders are even; the chest and abdomen are centered. Head remains in line with neck and shoulders (do not tilt or drop it). (Observe legs in Figure 7.)

*Walking Step Space*: Notice that the length of a step is about one and a half times the length of your foot. The feet are in the diagonal of an imaginary oblong which is one length of your foot in width. Each foot is in line with its hip, so that the body is completely centered. (Fig. 6)

Traveling in the Walking Step: always go from the Empty Step (from which you find your proper spacing and balance) into the Walking Step itself. (Fig. 8, 1 to 2)

Advancing in the Walking Step: Bring the back leg from its position, close to the other one: make the foot loose. (Fig. 8, 2 to 3) Place it forward in the Empty Step, then transfer weight onto it. You are in the Walking Step on the other leg. (Fig. 8, 3 to 4).

Retreating (going backward) in the Walking Step: When you bring the forward leg close to the one on which the weight rests, make the foot loose. Then place it backward in line with your hip; do not take the weight off the forward leg, which has all the weight.

The entire body is always on a slant in the completed Walking Step, as in Figure 7.

These positions occur on either side.

9. *Raised Leg position*: When a leg is raised and *straightened*, the knee must not be *stiffened*. The lower part of the leg is in line with the thigh. (Fig. 9)

When a leg is raised and *bent*, then the knee is kept high. There are two examples for this position: (a) When lower leg is held quite high, and thigh is held at an angle to a body with bent knee high. (The foot is always flexed inward, see 10 below.) (Fig. 120). (b) When leg movement is in transition; then the lower part of leg moves downward and the knee bends at an acute angle, while the foot is always loose (see 5 above).

10. *Foot position (Chiao Fa)*: (a) Foot is extended and turned inward, with instep and *toes* leading (called *T'i Chiao*). (Fig. 101). (b) Foot is flexed and turned inward, with *heel* leading (called *Teng Chiao*). (Fig. 120)

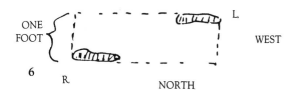

Toes are pointing west. This is the Walking Step Space. Feet are one foot apart, separated in length by one and a half feet, more or less.

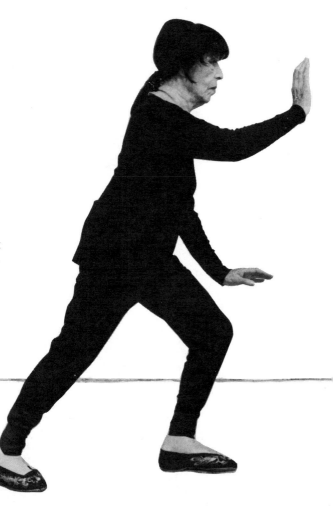

7

*11.* *Movements of Feet—Toes and Heel*: Take the basic stance with feet parallel and apart with knees bent. Pivoting on right toes, move right heel to the right. Straighten left knee. Keep right knee bent; try not to show shift of weight. Your torso is turned to west. You are now in a T-Step, with toed-in position. This occurs on either foot. (Fig. 10)

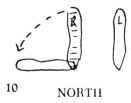

10    NORTH

The shaded foot is the moving foot.

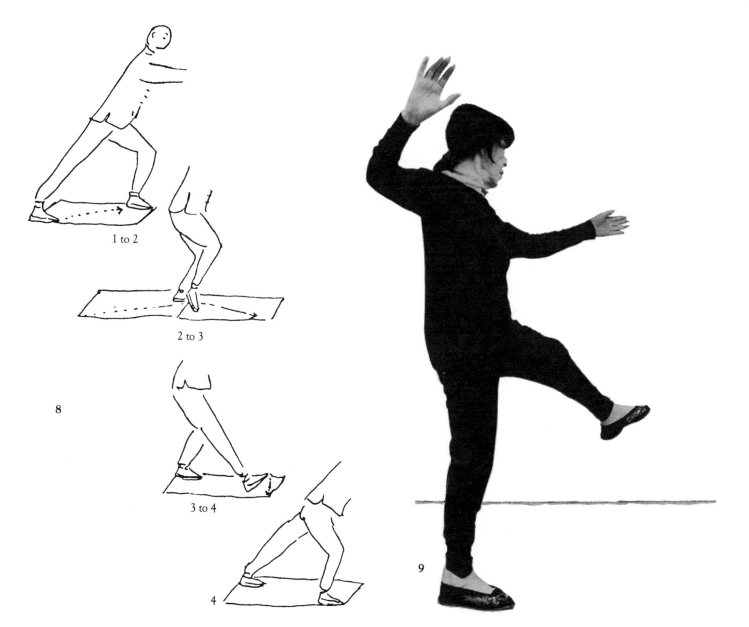

1 to 2

2 to 3

8

3 to 4

4

9

Take the Seated Position (as in 7 above) with feet apart twice the length of your foot and toes out at a slight angle. Turn right toe inward slightly, making right foot parallel to left foot; then move right heel outward, getting into a T-Step or toed-in position. Keep right knee bent with weight on it. Straighten left knee. This occurs on either foot. There are always *two* movements on one foot, when the foot moves from a seated position. (Fig. 11, 1 and 2)

12. *The Toe-Heel-Heel Step*: This is a combination of the T-Step and the basic stance with feet parallel and apart. Take the Walking Step position with left leg forward, left knee bent, body slanting forward, right leg straight. Turn left toes inward, keep weight on left leg with its bent knee, straighten hips out so that torso is erect. Then move right heel inward and bend right knee; weight is still on the left side. This movement makes the feet parallel. Now move left heel outward keeping weight on left leg with its bent knee; straighten right knee, and now you are in the T-step on the other side.

From this step, move into the Empty Step: with weight on left leg with its bent knee, raise right toes and keep right heel lightly on ground; foot is flexed, and knee is straight. Feet are parallel, although right ankle is flexed (otherwise right foot would be in toed-in position). You are seated on left with bent knee. (Fig. 58)

Level of body must be kept even during these changes.

This step is only done from left to right; weight remains on left during movement.

13. *The Hand position* or *Palm method* (*Chang Fa*) and *the Hand Form*: The hands are held loosely, knuckles and joints are not stiffened or tightened. From the position where your arms hang down, with loose elbows, note the hand form. The hands curve inward slightly, and the palm is curved. (Fig. 12)

Hands facing outside or away from body or upward are yang. (Figure 44) Hands facing inward or toward body or downward are yin. (Left hand, Figure 23) When palm faces to right or left of body, with fingers forward or upward, it is called Standing Palm (with an element of yin). (Right hand, Figure 100)

14. *The Fist position* (*Ch'üan Fa*): Close fingers lightly. Fold thumb over second and third fingers. Wrist is generally straight with a fisted hand. Elbows are dropped, that is, they point downward. Fist is tensed only on *quick* action.

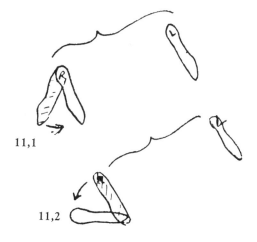

11,1

11,2

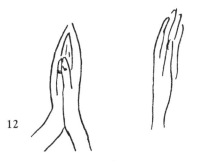

12

15.  *The Finger position*: Fingers are generally held rather close together. In some Forms the fingers are spread wide and apart from each other, as in Figure 13. In one Form, the Paw (*Chua*) or Grasping position, the finger, tips are close together grasping the thumb. The tip of the thumb touches the last joints of the fingers. Wrist is bent and the hand knuckles are bent. In this position, fingers always point to the floor. Finger tips must be directed correctly downward (concentration of energy in tips). (Right hand, Figure 32)

16.  *The Wrist position*: (a) Wrists are straightened so that hand and arms make a straight line. (Fig. 55) (b) Wrists are bent so that hand can face in many directions, at right angles to arm. (Fig. 44) (c) Wrists bend sideways: stretch arm forward with hand facing inward; move hand so that finger tips point diagonally downward, or diagonally upward; this is bending the wrist sideways. (Fig. 48)

17.  *Shoulder and Elbow position*: The shoulders must be controlled so that they do not push the movement; all strength comes from spine, not shoulders. Shoulders must be kept in *place*, not forward or pulled up. The elbows are kept low. When shoulders are loose and low, it is possible to control arm movement. When elbows are pointed outward or raised out of their natural position, then the shoulders are pulled forward out of place. (Fig. 24)

18.  *Waist position*: The waist is an important hinge, which must be loose and relaxed, but not slack. You must not press down into it. The torso lifts up from it. It is as "active as a cartwheel." When the waist can turn, the spine is flexible. The waist and spine control the exact position of the coccyx. If correct, they pull the buttocks in; when stiff, the back goes out "like a mountain peak." Hips must be kept level. (Fig. 216)

19.  *Eyes*: The eyes, unless directed to move with the hands, look forward and down at a diagonal (in relation to where the head is) with a quiet, easy, but steady gaze. "The eye is the cottage of the spirit."

20.  *Mouth and Tongue position*: Mouth must be kept lightly shut. The tip of tongue touches upper palate, behind teeth. The mouth is thus kept moist. "Saliva is sweet dew for cultivating life."

21.  *Breathing*: Breathe naturally, through the nose. The Forms will make you breathe deeply at certain times.

22.  *Body*: The body must be held "as steady as a mountain," and must feel "as light as a bird's feather."

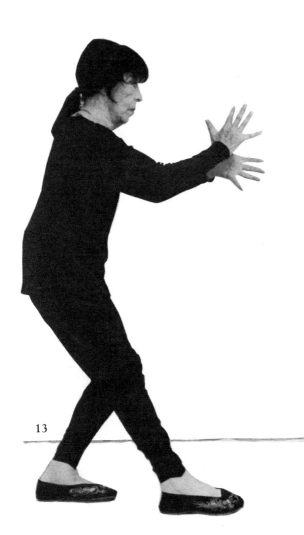

13

23.  *Stepping position*: The steps must be evenly paced and rhythmically exact as is "the walk of a cat." The toes of the forward foot must be directed exactly toward the angle of the designated design; for example, on stepping in the Walking Step toward the west, the toes of the forward foot must point exactly west.

*24. Shifting of Weight:* In the process of shifting your weight from one leg to the other, you must move so that the level of the head (torso and hips) remains the same. In changing position from one leg which is bent, to the other leg which is straight, the action is smooth and flowing. This is done by controlling the knee bend changes. (Fig. 14)

*25. Hand Circling and Wrist Rotation:* The circles, or parts of circles, that the hands describe in some of the movements are an extremely important element in the consideration of t'ai-chi ch'üan as a circular exercise. (1) Raise right arm forward shoulder high, with loose elbow, and bend wrist, pointing fingers upward with palm facing outward. (2) Circle hand outward to right; then bend hand downward making palm face inward. (3) Then circle over to the left and then upward with palm still facing inward, so that fingers point upward. (4) Turn palm outward, and it is once again in the starting position. Try to keep arm still, while the hand is moving. Do these movements with the left hand. Then circle both hands at the same time. Reverse the circle, making an inward rotation. (Fig. 15)

*26. Basic Tempo, Variations, and Synchronized Movements:* Control of tempo is essential for the proper synchronization of the Forms and patterns. The tempo with which you start the exercise is the basic one, the first movement of Form 1. When there is a variation, it is always *slower* than the basic tempo. In many Forms the arms will have to arrive at a given position at the same moment, although one may have to cover a larger space. Example: Raise your left arm forward, shoulder high, and raise your right arm up vertically. Both arms are to arrive at a low position along your side at the same moment. The right arm has farther to go, move it downward in the basic tempo. The left arm has a smaller space to travel, it therefore must move more slowly. This principle always holds: slow up the movement which has less space to traverse and must arrive at a given position, to coincide with a movement which has a greater distance to go.

*27. The Essence of the Motion:* The quality of the movement must never be strained. It is the control of movement, not the extent to which it can go, that gives both strength and softness at the same time.

*28. A Reserve of Energy:* The energy used must never be excessive or deficient; the first exhausts and the second delays development. In the process of learning, it is better to *underdo* than *overdo*. With properly guided energy you can feel "held together" and light at the same time. In action never strain at the joints. At every moment in the exercise you must have a reserve of energy and of movement which you know can be expanded at any moment.

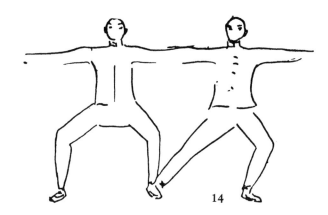

14

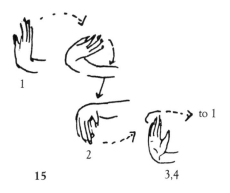

15

1. Read the directions out loud before you study each new sequence, but do *not* talk while you move. Let your mind direct you, so that you anticipate each movement as you act on it.

2. Give yourself enough time to learn to practice. Try to do the exercise regularly each day . Do not do too much at one time.

3. Each section carefully done will contribute to your well-being. You will never be impatient if you keep this in mind.

4. You must proceed slowly and accurately. Learn, relearn, and check what you do. When you practice, do everything three times: (1) to learn; (2) to correct and remember; and (3) very importantly, to experience the unity of what you do, and to capture its spirit.

5. Even when you have to stop in order to remember a sequence, try to hold the movement suspended, not frozen, as if you were a suddenly stopped motion picture.

6. If you remember that a light, even, flowing movement is essential for the feeling of calmness, you will more easily attain it. The idea of calmness will give you smooth movement; the smooth movement will give you calmness. Also remember that the Forms and patterns themselves, weaving into each other as they do structurally, will develop this essential quality, make you acquire it, since form and its function (of tranquility) are inextricably one.

7. Each time you start to practice, stand quietly for a few seconds. Fix your gaze steadily and lightly on the floor, at least ten feet away. Think of a slowly flowing river. This helps to eliminate outside problems and thoughts, and puts you in the mood for study.

8. Divide the units into parts; study each separately. Always organize the parts into their larger units and practice them as a flowing sequence. Distinguish between simultaneous and consecutive action. Do not omit the smaller details, such as moving a heel, toe, or hand, as each must be considered as a movement, complete in itself and as necessary to the structure as is the smallest part of a piece of complicated machinery.

9. Do not overwork a tiny part . Each unit must contain a light and strong movement; a leg, arm, and body movement, so that you benefit at each practice session from the activity of exercising the entire body.

10. Do everything lightly and without anxiety. Do not confuse lack  of anxiety with lack of effort or industriousness. You must make an effort to direct yourself with will. Light in action and deep in mind will result from effort with understanding.

11. Don't be hasty. Move slowly. No matter how much effort you put into practicing, you will feel enriched because of the vital Forms and the easy, calm process of the movement.

12. Refer to Basic Positions frequently.

13. Associate the names of the Forms with the patterns that go with them. You will then understand how complete a unit each Form is; how the yin-yang elements are balanced; how the Solid and Empty are dynamically related to each other; how the structural themes merge; and how they vary. You will begin to comprehend the subtlety of the whole composition mentally, physically, and aesthetically.

14. Notice: (1) how you warm up gradually; (2) how you develop strength and power as you practice; (3) that your breathing remains quiet and easy; (4) that the heart beat is not accelerated; (5) that you can maintain an easy calmness while learning; (6) that when you complete your daily practice, you have a sensation of well-being and tranquility.

15. To facilitate the understanding of the illustrations in terms of their moving directions, stand in front of a mirror, holding them in front of you, face out. You will see the image as moving in the direction you are to take. Where illustrations contain arrows, they indicate how the movements will proceed to the next position.

**Explanatory Notes**

*1. Space Directions:* Directions are given in terms of the compass: north, east, south, west, and the diagonals northeast, northwest, southeast, southwest. This method simplifies the delineation of space and keeps the text clear as to the difference between the sides of the body (right, left, front, back) and the sides of space.

Facing the North Star, you know that east is at your right, west at your left, and south behind you. This same principle is used for the directions of the spatial patterns, except that here we disregard the star's true directions. You must consider north that side of your room toward which you face to begin the exercise; then east is the right side of the room, west is the left side, and south is the back wall. These directions with North as the front I have changed from the recent Chinese way, which has South as the front. North was the *original direction*.

The illustrations are drawn with north as the point of reference. Look at them as you look at a photographic image. Therefore north is at the lower side of the diagram, toward which you face to begin. It will not be difficult to orient yourself to this concept of space. When you are actually in action, you feel the directions at eye level.

The floor pattern in space (the movement of the feet) is designed so as to cover more space toward the west than toward the east of the starting position. In the diagram, the dotted lines indicate the limit of space that you will traverse when you do the complete exercise. Therefore note the starting position (the arrow pointing north), east of the center of your room, in Figure 16. The exercise ends in exactly the same place at which it begins: see the Footchart at the end of this book.

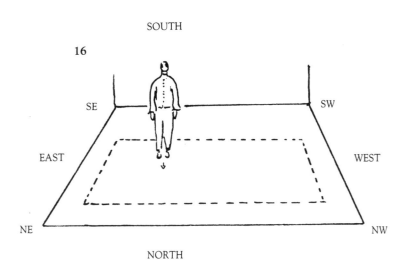

Space-Directions

2. *Names of Forms:* It is necessary to keep the standard names of the Forms, even though their meaning in English seems obscure. Though the names are not consistent as to motivation, they all have significance. Some are technically graphic and describe physical movement, as does Brush Knee Twist Step. Some indicate what the movement is, as rendered in Self-Defense, as in Parry, Obstruct, Punch. Others are derived from concepts or associations (but are not pantomimic). These, as in Hand Strums the Lute, suggest that the movement is like that of the particular image named.

There are some that have metaphysical significance such as Seven Stars, which may refer to the Big Dipper or, as some believe, to the seven openings of head and heart. The Bird and Snake imply wit, intelligence, and consciousness. (See page 173)

Other terms are metaphorical, as in Carry Tiger, Push Mountain; the tiger stands for lungs, or respiration, and is yin in quality. Perhaps The

38  Stork Flaps its Wings is so named because the movement activates that part of the body known as the Dove's Tail in ancient times. (It is an inch below the apex of the ensiform cartilage. See Figure 17.)

For our purposes it is best to accept the names as terms with which to identify the various structures. It is necessary to remember them in order to appreciate the composition as a whole, and eventually to understand their significance as they relate to movement.

*3. Division into Series (I-VI):* Although the division of the 108 Forms into six series has been made to simplify the process of learning, it has not been done arbitrarily. Each series has structural meaning, as well as physical and psychological aspects. The developments and variations in the designs and themes of each series are distinctly vital in balancing the creative unity of the whole. Nevertheless, they are not to be thought of separately, except perhaps when learning them. There is no physical division, however, no cessation of movement either between the parts, or at any moment of the exercise.

*4. Method of Classification:* Since the Forms *are* the exercise, the directions for executing them are separated according to their structure. It is to be assumed that each part continues from the preceding one; therefore it has not been necessary to say, "Continue from the preceding position" each time. And, to reiterate, since the exercise does not stop at any point, each unit, no matter how small or large, is linked to the next one.

There are consecutive and simultaneous movements. And there are places where parts of the body are inactive, when other parts are active. Necessarily, the written directions have to isolate the various movements. Generally speaking, a complete part is described, with the legs', arms' and body's action analyzed in a single paragraph. "At the same time," "simultaneously" indicate the synchronized action of several parts of the body. Unless otherwise stated, the action is consecutive; or if not mentioned at all, quiescence of the unmentioned part is to be assumed. These are to be carefully watched: stillness and movement, and consecutive and simultaneous action. The ultimate harmony of t'ai-chi ch'üan lies in the relationship of consecutive flowing movement, the fleeting second of simultaneous completeness of movement, and the utter immovability of that part which must be quiet.

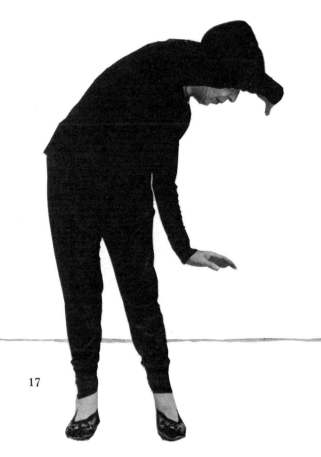

17

# Part Two:

*The Exercise-Art of T'ai-Chi Ch'üan*

## SERIES 1

**Form 1. Beginning Form of T'ai-Chi Ch'üan**  *T'ai-Chi Ch'üan Ch'i Shih*
Face north. Stand tall, with head straight and shoulders low. With feet parallel, separate them so that the space between them is equal to the length of your foot. This is your basic stance: feet parallel and apart. Your legs are on a perfect perpendicular. Place your arms down along your sides, with wrists straight and palms facing the rear (south). Look ahead of you on the floor about ten feet away. Feet centered, easy, quiet. Mouth is shut lightly, not tightly, and must remain so throughout the entire exercise. (Fig. 18)

Raise both arms forward and up to shoulder level; wrists remain straight and are shoulder width apart. This simple movement establishes the tempo that you must maintain throughout the exercise; it focuses your mind and makes you feel light and calm. (Fig. 19)

Draw arms in toward shoulders by bending both elbows downward bending wrists at the same time. Palms face the floor. (Fig. 20)

Lift both hands so that palms face north. Then move arms downward to the sides of the thighs, keeping wrists bent with palms facing floor. At the same time as the arms move, bend both knees, keeping back straight and buttocks tucked in. (Fig. 21)

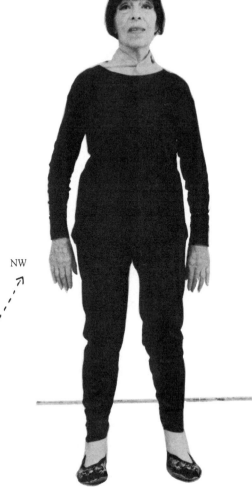

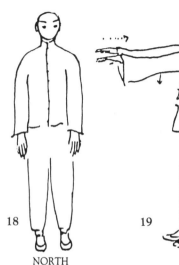

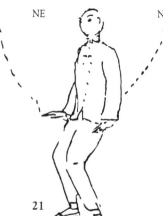

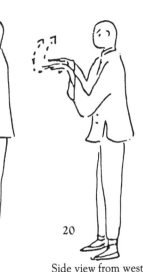

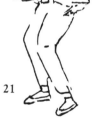

18
NORTH

19

20

21

Side view from west

Keeping palms facing floor, move right hand so that fingers point northeast, and move left hand so that fingers point northwest; shift weight to right leg all at the same time.

Raise both arms straight up in their diagonals, with fingers pointing upward, palms out. Right palm faces northeast and left faces northwest; both wrists come to slightly higher than shoulder level. At the same time as arms move, move left leg directly north, shifting all your weight onto the right leg with its already-bent knee. Straighten left kneee and place heel lightly on floor with toes upraised—this is a flexed foot. Arms and legs arrive in position together. (Fig. 22)

Hold this leg position (called Empty Step, see page 28). Both arms move at the same time: move right arm, with palm facing outward, to the center in front of chest about six inches away; turn left palm inward, moving arm in the front so that palm is toward the forehead about six inches away. Left elbow is shoulder height; right elbow points downward. (Fig. 23)

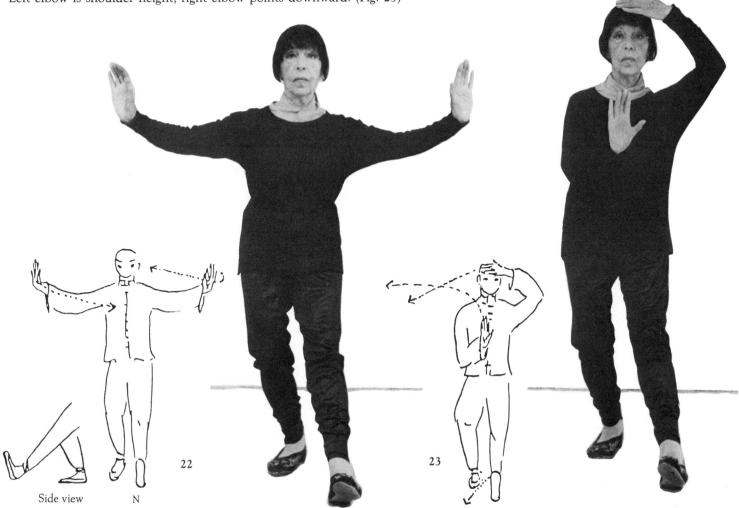

22

Side view      N

23

## Form 2. Grasping the Bird's Tail *Lan Ch'ueh Wei*

First

Turn toes of left foot toward the east, by pivoting on the heel. Place left foot on floor and bend knee at the same time, while straightening the right knee. Weight is on the left leg and torso is turned to northeast. Feet are in the T-step position (see page 28) with left toes pointing east and right toes north.

As you place left toes to the east move both arms. Right arm, fingers leading, moves to the east, left arm lowers to shoulder level; right palm faces north, and left palm faces south. (Fig. 24 sequence)

Move right leg toward the east, straightening knee, and place heel on floor with foot flexed (Empty Step). Weight is on left leg. At the same time

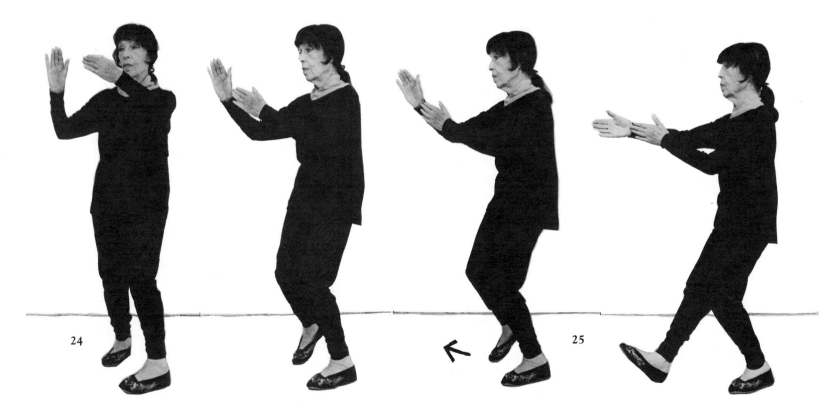

24

25

extend right arm to the east so that its pulse is at the point of left finger tips. Both elbows are loose and curved downward. Hands are at chest level. Left fingers do not touch right pulse. (Fig. 25)

Keeping the relationship of hands the same, draw both arms in toward body at chest level, bending both elbows downward and slightly out with right wrist nine inches from chest. Do not move legs.

Turn right palm up and left palm down. As you move hands, angle left hand so that it is at a right angle to right wrist, raising left elbow. Now left elbow points north. (Fig. 26)

## Form 3. Grasping the Bird's Tail    *Lan Ch'üeh Wei*

Second

Transfer weight onto right leg, bending right knee and straightening left knee. Weight is forward and body is on a diagonal line from head to left heel. Buttocks are tucked in and hips are centered. At the same time stretch right arm to the northeast shoulder high straightening wrist and elbow. Keep left fingers near right wrist. (Fig. 27)

Circle both arms horizontally, shoulder high, going from northeast to east, to south; send right elbow downward, bending right wrist so that palm faces upward. Turn right fingers to point southwest at the end of this horizontal circling. Left arm is adjusted to the movement of right arm, because left finger tips always remain near right pulse. Right elbow is down and left elbow points northeast.

As the same time as you bend elbow from southeast, shift weight back onto left leg by bending its knee, and straighten right leg, flexing right foot (Empty Step). (Fig. 28)

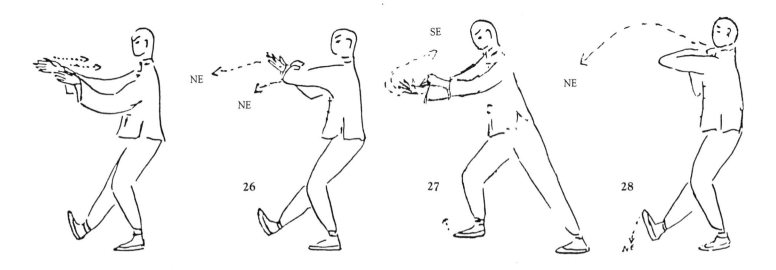

26    27    28

**Form 4. Grasping the Bird's Tail** *Lan Ch'üeh Wei*

Third

Pivot on right heel, to northeast, flexing foot. At the same time, raise right arm, with palm leading, arcing upward head high and then down toward the northeast, straightening arm as you do so. Stop in position when right wrist is slightly above shoulder height; palm faces northeast.

As you are approaching this last position with the right arm, place toes on floor, bend right knee, placing weight on right leg, and straighten left knee. Then bend right wrist and lower hand, making fingers point downward. As hand bends down, place all the fingers over the thumb in grasping position (see Fig. 29). Right arm does not move out of its position as hand bends down. Left fingers remain near right pulse with palm facing your face; left wrist is straight and arm is curved. (Fig. 29)

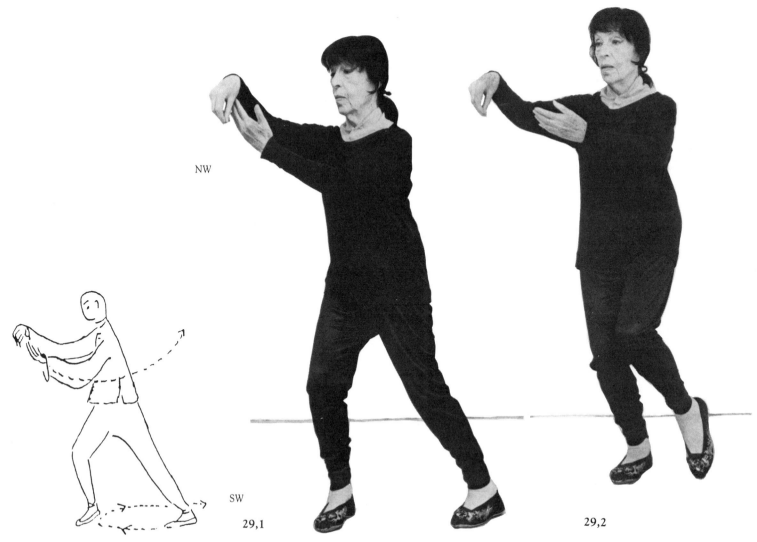

NW

SW

29,1

29,2

Hold weight on right leg with its bent knee. Draw left foot with loose ankle close to right, without touching floor with left toes. Then move left leg backward to southwest diagonal in the Walking Step Space (see page 30; observe the arrows for the feet in Fig. 29). Straighten left knee and place foot parallel to right foot; each foot is in its own track as in the Walking Step. Weight is on right leg, and body is on a diagonal slant toward northeast. As left leg moves, move left arm, with palm toward your face, in a downward curve in toward the body, within eight inches of chest. Then raise it up and out toward the northwest, shoulder-high. Right arm does not move. Torso is being centered north. (Fig. 30)

Pivoting on left heel, turn toes toward the northwest. Place weight on left leg and bend knee to equal bend of right knee. Now your weight is even on both legs. Body is turned to northwest. Feet are separated by a distance equal to twice the length of your foot. Your back is straight. As left foot moves, turn left palm to face northwest, with fingers pointing upward. Now both arms are on the same level, with wrists slightly higher than shoulder level. Right arm is extended toward northeast, and left arm toward northwest; right toes point to northeast, and left toes to northwest. Right hand is in grasping position, and left wrist is bent with palm northwest. (Fig. 31)

Movements of Head and Eyes for Form 5.

Take position as in Figure 29. Look at left palm; keep looking at it as hand moves down, and then up to northwest. Turn head from right to left side, but do not bend it downward when eyes look downward. The top of head is kept level as head moves from right to left side. When left palm turns to northwest, you will then be looking at the back of hand. (Fig. 31 shows the sequence of the Single Whip)

Eyes, arm, legs, and body movements are synchronized.

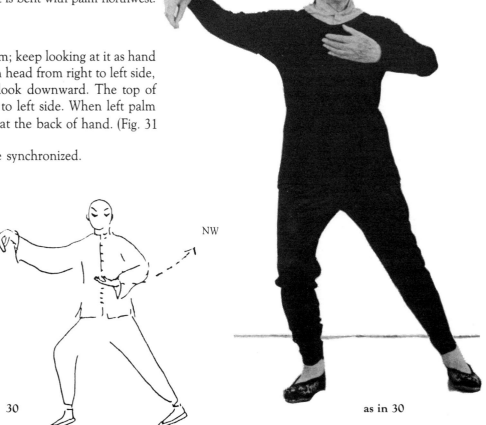

NW

30

as in 30

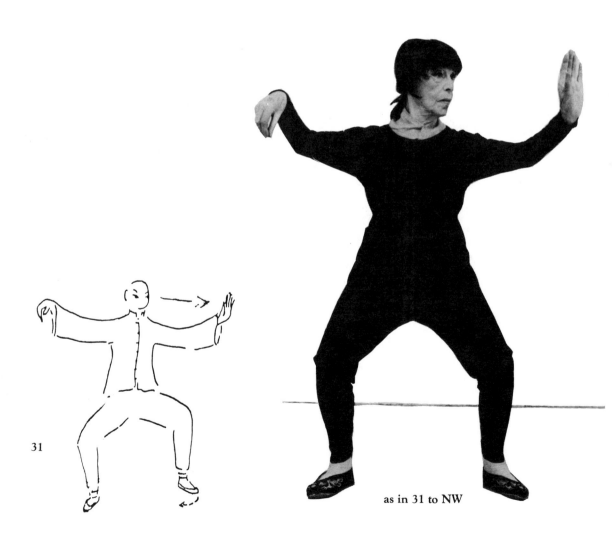

31

as in 31 to NW

## Form 6. Raise Hands and Step Up     *T'i Shou Shang Shih*

Adding weight on left leg with its bent knee, turn toes of left foot to north; straighten right knee, which turns torso north. At the same time, turn left palm upward, straightening wrist; fingers point to northwest. You are now looking at left palm. Do not tilt torso. (Fig. 33)

Bend head so that left ear is directed toward left shoulder. Now the face is north, on a slant, with chin centered. As the head moves, open right hand and turn palm upward. Look at right palm, but do not move head. You are now looking obliquely toward the right. Right fingers point northeast. (Fig. 34)

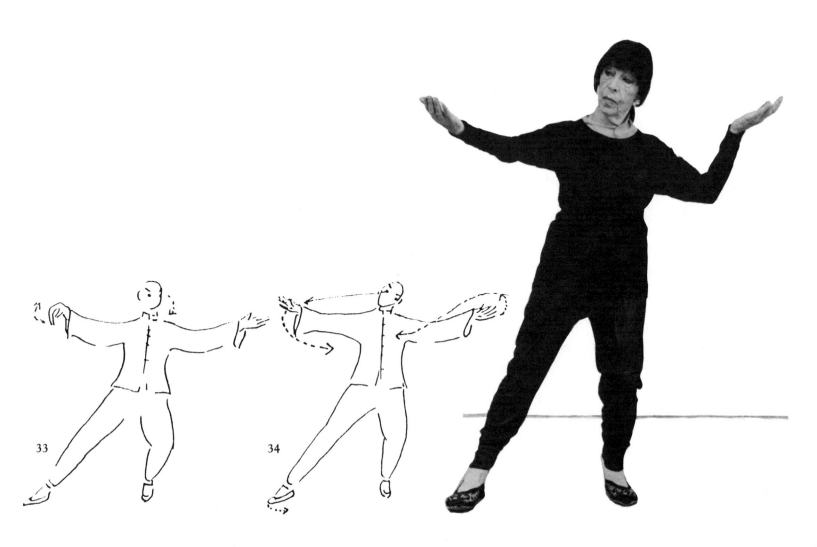

33          34

Turn right toes north. Bend right knee and straighten left leg. Place weight forward on right leg; turn head to north and straighten torso toward north. Then, bend the torso forward north as both arms move: bring right arm in a curve forward, chest high, fifteen inches from body, and move left hand, with palm turned toward northeast, directly to inner curve of the right elbow. Left elbow points downward, right elbow is chest high. (Fig. 35) As arms are completing the movement, place left foot parallel and apart, from the right foot, in your basic stance (Fig. 18), bending left knee. Now both knees are evenly bent. The back is curved; torso is front; weight is equal on both legs. (Fig. 36)

Raise body to an upright position and straighten knees. At the same time, lift right curved arm to a position just above forehead, and lower left arm with palm down to front of left thigh. Wrist is bent and fingers point north. Arms and body finish together. (Fig. 37) Then, as a *separate* movement, turn the right hand to face palm upward, bending wrist.

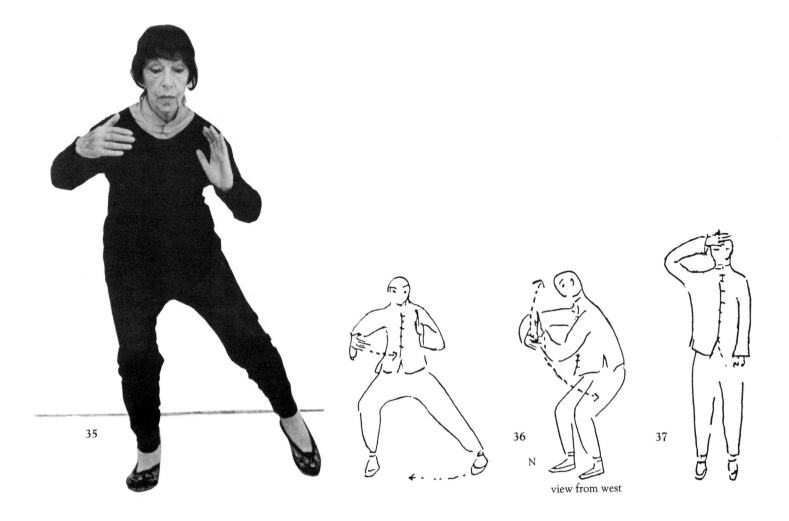

35

36

N

view from west

37

## Form 7. White Stork Flaps its Wings    *Pai Hao Liang Ch'ih*

Do not move right arm from its place near top of forehead for the next sequences.

Bend torso forward down and, at the same time, move left arm away from thigh so that it is perpendicular to floor, palm facing floor, hand is knee level. (Fig. 38)

Keep arms in same relative positions. Twist torso to west, keeping body low. Arms move with body. Fingers of left hand point west. Left arm is close to body. (Fig. 39)

Lift torso up erect, remaining turned to west. At the same time, bring straight left arm up shoulder high. Left wrist is bent; palm faces west with fingers pointing upward. Head and torso are turned west; knees are straight. Eyes look at left hand. (Fig. 40)

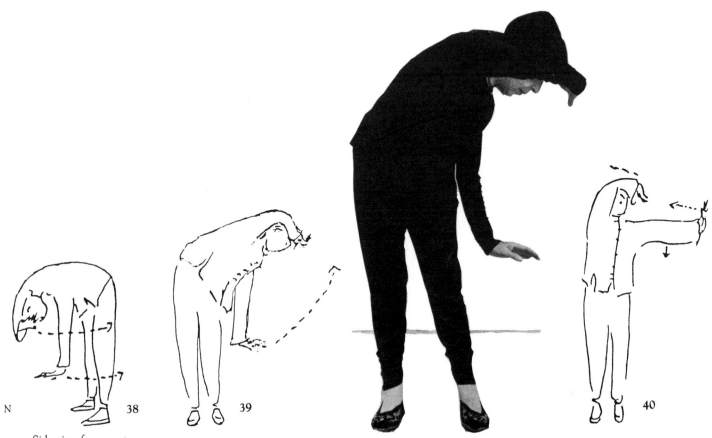

N            38                    39                                                    40

Side view from west

50  Turn torso to north. As you do this, bend left elbow and bring left hand to center of forehead, with palm north, so that fingers point to right finger tips. Right palm faces north. Finger tips do not touch each other; hands are a fist length away from forehead. The legs are straight. (Fig. 41)

Bend both knees, keeping back straight. At the same time as you bend knees, move both hands: bend the wrists and turn hands so that palms face diagonally front-downward. Keep hands at forehead level. At the same time as hands move, press elbows diagonally forward so that right elbow points northeast and left points northwest, both being at shoulder level. Make this movement with strength and hardness. Feel the tensed contraction in muscles of upper arms. This contrasts with the light, intrinsic movement you have been using up to now. Feel as if you were holding or pressing the upper half of a ball between elbows and hands. Knees and hands move together. (Fig. 42)

### Form 8. Brush Knee Twist Step     *Lou Hsi Niu Pu*
Right Side
Keeping weight on right leg with its bent knee, shift right heel to east: this movement turns torso to face west, releasing the weight from left leg; raise left heel off floor. As body and legs turn to west, turn right palm inward toward forehead and turn left palm outward. Then circle left arm outward and downward, and move right arm down while left hand goes under right as right hand circles above left wrist. By this time you are facing west. Both hands are ten inches away from chest. Right palm faces south with fingers pointing west. Elbow is down. Left wrist is bent, with fingers north and palm west. (Fig. 43)

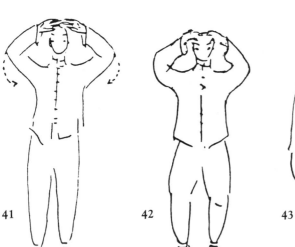

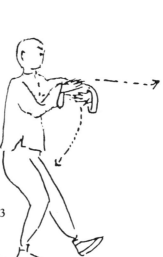

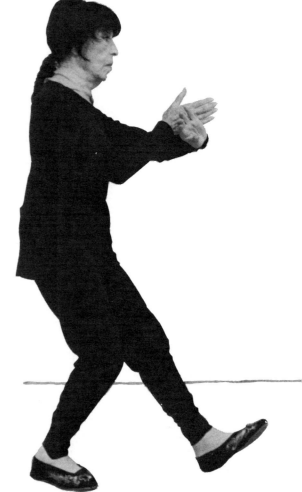

41          42          43

Moving left leg west, place heel in Empty Step Space with straight knee and flexed foot. Transfer weight onto left leg, bending left knee, and straightening right knee. Body slants on a diagonal toward west. As you step west both arms move: move right arm to west in line with right shoulder, turning palm to face west with fingers pointing upward . At the same time, circle left arm with bent wrist downward, and place left hand in front of left thigh. Palm faces floor, with fingers pointing west. (Fig. 44)

### Form 9. Hand Strums the Lute    *Shou Hui P'i-P'a*
Shift weight back onto right leg, bending right knee, and at the same time, straighten left knee and flex foot. As legs move, both arms move: bring right arm inward nine inches from face, keeping right palm facing west with fingers pointing up. Move left hand upward and place finger tips at right pulse. Left palm faces inward toward the heart. Arms and legs move at the same time. (Fig. 45)

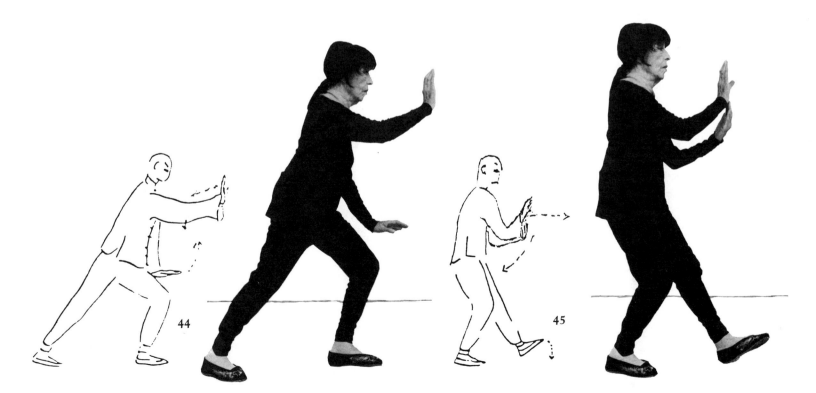

44                                    45

**Form 10. Brush Knee Twist Step**    *Lou Hsi Niu Pu*

Same as Form 8, Figure 44.

Transfer weight to left foot in the Walking Step (see page 30): left knee is bent, right knee is straight, and body slants on a diagonal forward. As you do this, move right arm west directly in line with right shoulder, turning palm to west with wrist shoulder high. At the same time, move left arm downward in front of left thigh with palm facing floor. Both arms and leg move and finish at the same time (Fig. 44)

Brush Knee Twist Step
On left side

Draw right foot with loose ankle to Empty Step, heel touching floor. At the same time both arms move: move left hand with fingers pointing west (palm is north) up to center, and move right hand (palm west) inward toward center, keeping wrist bent with fingers pointing south. Move left hand above right wrist. Both hands meet in center, ten inches away from chest. (This position is opposite to that of Figure 43.)

Move right leg forward west. Straightening knee and flexing foot, touch heel to floor in the Walking Step Space. Then transfer weight onto right foot, bending right knee and straightening left knee. Body slants forward on a diagonal. At the same time as legs move, both arms move: move left arm toward the west in line with left shoulder, turning palm to west, with wrist shoulder high; move right arm with bent wrist down in front of right thigh, palm facing floor with fingers pointing west. Both arms and legs move together. (This position is opposite to that of Figure 44.)

Brush Knee Twist Step
On right side

Draw left foot with loose ankle in toward right foot without touching floor. At the same time both arms move: move right hand up with fingers pointing west (palm is south) and move left hand inward toward the center of chest keeping wrist bent, fingers pointing north. Right hand moves above left wrist. Both hands meet in center, ten inches away from chest. (Fig. 46, 1)

Move left leg forward west. Straightening knee and flexing foot, touch heel to floor in the Empty Step Space. Then transfer weight onto left foot, bending left knee and straightening right knee. Body slants on a diagonal west. As you step west both arms move: move right arm west directly in line with right shoulder, turning palm to face west with wrist shoulder high, and move left arm downward in front of left thigh with palm facing floor, fingers pointing west. Both arms and legs move and finish at the same time. (Fig. 46, 2)

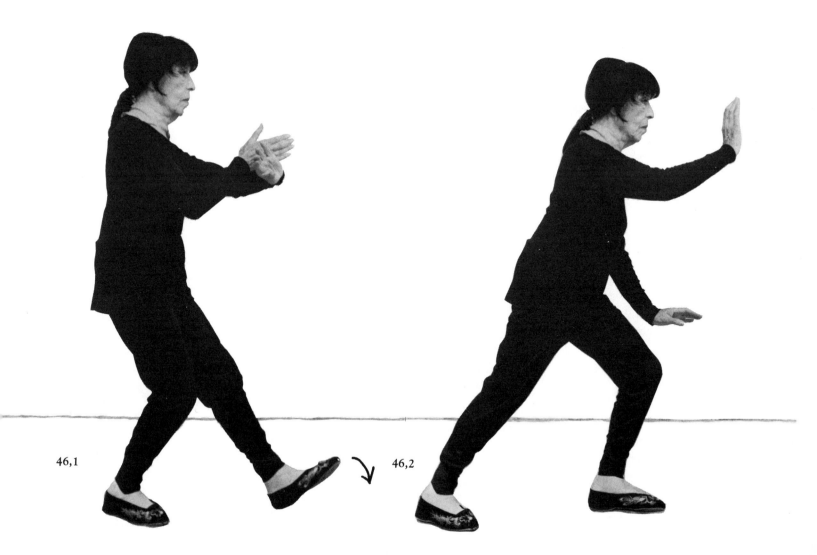

46,1

46,2

**Form 11. Hand Strums the Lute**     *Shou Hui P'i-P'a*

On left side

Keeping left knee bent, move the right foot and place it parallel and apart
from left in your basic stance: both knees are bent and body is straight.
Both arms move at the same time as right leg. With palm west, move left
arm up ten inches from face, while you move right hand inward, turning
palm inward, and place right finger tips near left pulse. Right palm faces
heart. (Fig. 47)

**Form 12. Step up, Parry, and Punch**     *Chin Pu Pan Lan Ch'ui*

Move left leg forward west, straightening knee and flexing foot. Touch
heel to floor in the Empty Step Space. Then transfer weight onto left foot,
bending left knee and straightening right knee. Body slants on a diagonal
west. At the same time, move both arms forward west in line with left
shoulder; turn left palm to north with fingers pointing west-downward.
Right fingers remain at left pulse: therefore, right palm turns to face south,
and right elbow points downward. (Fig. 48)

Shift weight back onto right leg, bending right knee, straightening left
knee, and flexing left foot (Empty Step). At the same time, both arms
move: draw right hand down toward right hip bone, closing it gradually,
so that when it reaches the hip, the hand is fisted lightly. Right elbow
points to north, right shoulder contracts, fist-palm is turned upward so
that knuckles point to floor. While right arm moves, angle left hand so
that fingers point west-upward. Do not move left arm out of its position.

Shift weight forward onto left leg, bending left knee and straightening
right knee. At the same time, both arms move: move right arm up west in
line with right shoulder, with fist-palm facing south, elbow straight. Move
left palm near inner side of right elbow; left wrist is bent with fingers
pointing upward. Arm movements and shifting of weight go together. (Figure
49 shows the sequence of the punch.)

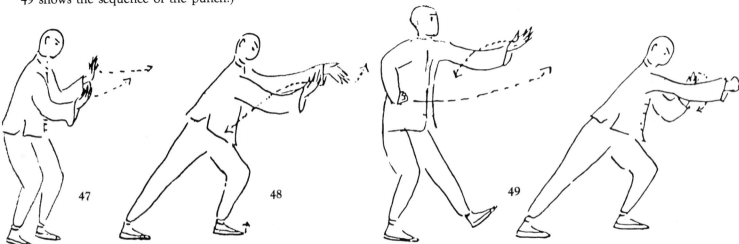

47                48                49

## Form 13. As If You Were Shutting a Door   *Ju Feng Szu Pi*

Do not move legs or torso. Move left hand under right arm to its outer side, and turn palm to face right elbow. (Fig. 50)

Shift weight back onto right leg, bending right knee, and straighten left knee, flexing left foot. At the same time, both arms move: bend right elbow bringing the right fist in toward left shoulder, opening the fist gradually so that palm faces left shoulder, and move left palm, facing inward, in to face right shoulder. Left arm is on the outside of right arm. Both elbows are bent downward and forearms are crossed on a diagonal.

At the same time both arms move: move right hand in front of right shoulder with palm facing it and move left in front of left shoulder with palm facing it. Elbows are bent downward, wrists are straight, and fingers point upward.

Then turn both palms to face west, keeping wrists straight and elbows down. All these arm movements are made as weight is shifted from left leg back to right leg with bent knee. (Fig. 51)

## Form 14. Carry Tiger To Mountain   *Pao Hu Kuei Shan*

Shift weight forward onto left leg, bending left knee and straightening right knee. At the same time, push both hands, which are facing west, forward shoulder high, to west, each arm in line with its shoulder: wrists are shoulder high, and body slants forward on a diagonal west. (Fig. 52)

Keep weight on left leg. Bend torso down, contracting pelvis, moving arms at same time, and lower arms so that palms face floor at knee level. Arms are perpendicular to floor. (Fig. 53)

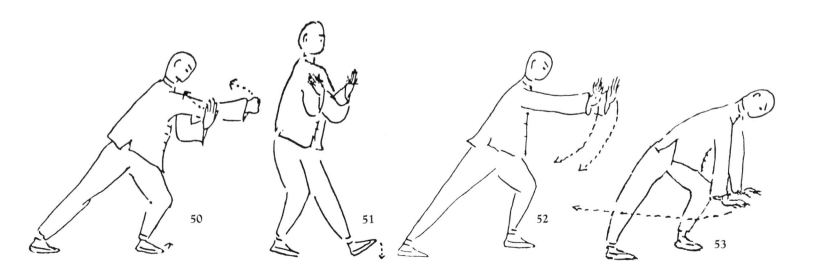

50    51    52    53

**Form 15. Cross Hands** *Shih Tzu Shou*

Turn right toes to north, and at the same time shift weight onto right leg, bending right knee and straightening left knee. With these movements, torso moves to north, still remaining bent over; do not lower head. At the same time as torso and right toes move, move right hand to right side of right leg, keeping palm down. Right fingers now point east. Left hand remains at left side; palm is down with fingers pointing west. (Fig. 54; opposite of Figure 217)

Gradually raise the torso to an upright position, bringing arms up sideways, shoulder high, straightening wrist. Then move them forward north, shoulder high. At same time, turn left toes north. (Fig. 55)

Keeping right knee bent, place left foot parallel to right and apart from it in your basic stance. Both knees are bent. At the same time as leg moves, bring both arms inward, crossing forearms diagonally: right forearm is on the outside of left forearm, left palm faces east on a slant, and right palm faces west on a slant. The V cross of the arms is just below chin level about eight inches away: elbows are high and back is straight. (Fig. 56)

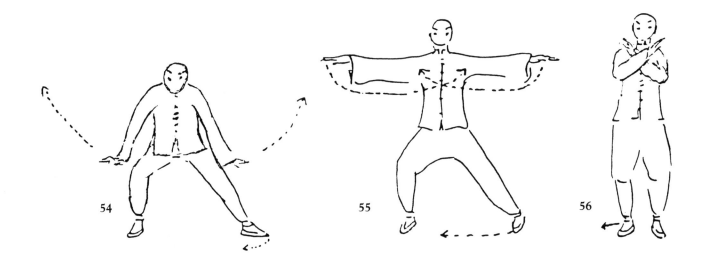

54          55          56

To northwest on right side

Move heel of right foot outward to southeast, keeping weight on right leg with its bent knee. This movement releases weight from left leg and turns torso to face northwest. (See Figure 129)

Move left leg to northwest, straightening knee and flexing foot. Place heel on floor in the Empty Step Space. Then transfer weight onto left foot, bending knee and straightening right knee. Body slants forward northwest. At the same time, both arms move: move right arm forward northwest in line with right shoulder, turning palm to face northwest, and move left arm with bent wrist downward in front of left thigh; fingers point northwest and palm is down. (Fig. 57)

Toe—Heel—Heel—Step

Keeping weight on left leg with its bent knee, move left toes inward to point northeast. Straighten torso. At the same time, both arms begin to move: move left hand upward with fingers leading, with elbow low at chest level and move right hand inward toward body. (Fig. 58, 1)

Keeping weight on left leg with its bent knee, move right heel inward, making right foot parallel to left, and bend right knee, so that toes of both feet point northeast. Weight is still on left leg and torso is straight. At the same time, continue to move both hands toward center of body, with left hand approaching right wrist. (Fig. 58, 2)

Keeping weight on left leg with its bent knee, move left heel outward to northwest. With this movement torso faces east and right knee straightens. Feet are now in T position (see page 31). At the same time, arms move: continue to move left hand to right wrist, with left fingers pointing southeast; right wrist is bent. (Fig. 58, 3)

Weight is still on left leg with its bent knee. Turning torso to face southeast, raise right toes off floor. At the same time, both arms move: move right arm with bent wrist toward front of chest and move left hand over right wrist. (Fig. 58,4)

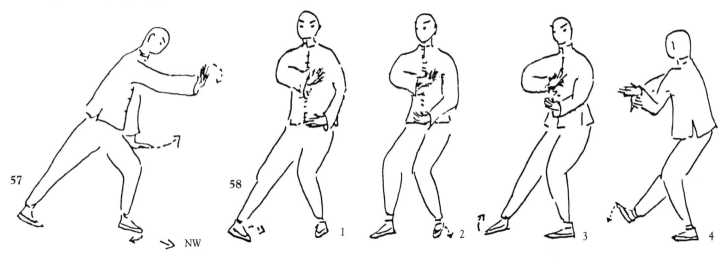

57    58    1    2    3    4    NW

Oblique Brush Knee Twist Step

To southeast on left side, position opposite to that of Figure 57..

Place right heel to southeast, in the Empty Step Space. Transfer weight onto right leg, bending right knee and straightening left knee. Body slants southeast on a diagonal. At the same time, both arms move: move left arm to southeast in line with left shoulder, turning palm out to face southeast; and move right hand down to front of right thigh, with palm facing floor and fingers pointing southeast.

## Form 17. Grasping the Bird's Tail *Lan Ch'üeh Wei*

First

Shift weight back onto left leg, bending knee, straightening right knee, and flexing right foot. At the same time, both arms move: bring right arm up to southeast, chest high, with palm facing northeast, and place left fingers at right pulse. (Figure 25—except that here you face the southeast diagonal instead of east.)

Keep the relationship of hands the same. Bending both elbows downward and slightly out, draw both arms inward toward body at chest level, nine inches away from it.

Turn right palm up and left palm down. As hands move, angle left hand so that it is at right angles to right wrist; therefore, left elbow points northeast. (Fig. 26, except that here you face southeast.)

Grasping the Bird's Tail
Second

Transfer weight onto the right leg, bending right knee and straightening left knee, with body on a slant diagonally toward southeast. As the same time as you do this, stretch right arm to the east, shoulder high, straightening elbow. Keep left fingers above right pulse. (Fig. 27, except that here you face southeast.)

Move both arms in a horizontal circle, shoulder high, from east to southeast, to south, to west. When arms reach south, bend right elbow downward and bend right wrist so that palm faces upward. Turn right fingers to point west at end of horizontal circling; left elbow points east. Left arm is adjusted to movement of right arm, because left fingers always remain near right pulse.

As you move arms from south, shift weight back onto left leg, bending left knee, and straighten right knee, flexing foot (Empty Step). (Fig. 28, except that here you face southeast.)

Third

Pivot on right heel, turning toes to east. At the same time, raise right arm with palm up arcing upward, head high, then down toward the east, straightening arm as you do so. Stop at a place where right wrist is slightly above shoulder height.

As you are approaching this last position, place toes on floor, bend right knee, placing weight on right leg, bend right wrist and lower right hand downward so that fingers point downward. As hand bends down, place all fingers close together over thumb as if grasping it. Right arm remains in its position when wrist bends and fingers move. Left fingers are still at right pulse, with palm toward the face. Left wrist is straight and arm is curved. (Fig. 29, except here the right hand and foot face directly east.)

## Form 18. The Single Whip    *Tan Pien*

Holding weight on right leg, draw left foot close to right—without touching floor. Continue to move left leg: place it in northwest diagonal in the Walking Step Space. Straighten left knee and place foot parallel to right foot. Body is on a diagonal slant toward the east. While moving left leg, move left arm in a downward curve, in toward the body, chest high. Continue to move it, raising arm upward toward the north. Arm is curved, palm faces upward toward the face. (Fig. 32, except that here the direction of the right hand and foot is east.)

Pivoting on left heel, turn toes toward north, at the same time bending left knee to equal bend of right knee. Weight is equal on both legs. Feet are separated by a distance equal to twice the length of the foot. Back is straight. As you move left foot, turn left hand to face palm north. Now both arms are on the same level; wrists are slightly higher than shoulder level. Right arm is toward east in grasping position, and left palm faces north. Right toes point east, and left toes point north. Body is turned to northeast. (Fig. 59)

Movements of Head and Eyes for Form 18

Look at left palm; keep eyes on it as arm moves to north. Turn head from right to left sides, but do not *bend* it downward when eyes look downward. The top of head is kept level as head turns. When left palm faces north eyes will then look at back of hand. (Fig. 32, except that here the final direction of the left hand and foot is north.) Eyes, head, arm, legs and body movements must be synchronized.

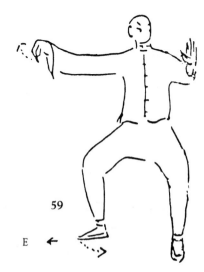

**59**

E ←

N

**Form 19. Fist Under Elbow**     *Chou Ti K'an Ch'ui*

Move right toes to point north and at the same time shift weight to left bent leg, straightening right knee. This movement turns torso north. Keep head facing north: arm moves with torso: left arm will be northwest, right arm will be northeast. As you shift weight, open right hand so that palm faces upward and right wrist is straight. Foot, weight, torso, and hand move together. (Fig. 60)

Move left toes to point west, keeping left knee bent with weight remaining on left. This movement turns torso (which is on a diagonal) west. At the same time as toes and torso move, turn left palm upward with straightened wrist. Both arms move with torso. Keep arms outstretched at shoulder level as torso faces toward west: left arm extends to southwest; right arm extends to northwest and both palms face up. (Fig. 61) During this action, the arms have remained at the "Single Whip" angle, diagonal to shoulders.

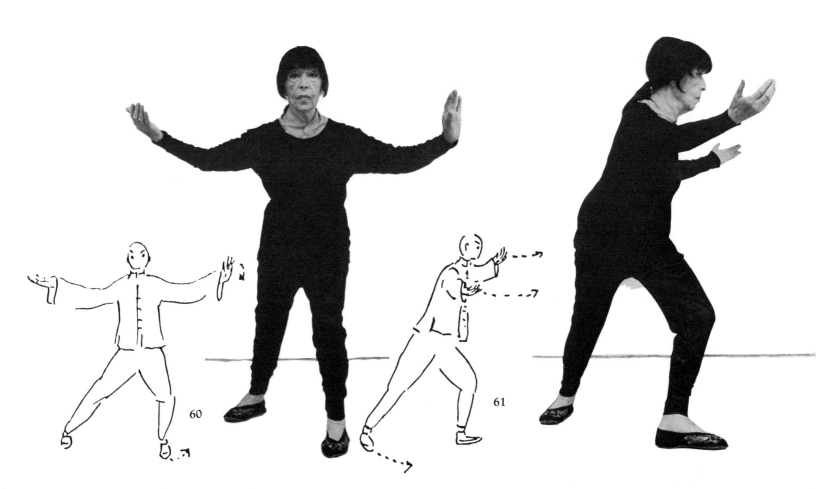

60

61

Hold weight on left leg, bend right knee, and then place right foot back to east in the Walking Step Space. Body remains on a slant toward west. While moving right leg, move both arms towards west, turning palms downward. Keep arms shoulder high. Hands with straight wrists are shoulder width apart. (Fig. 62)

Shift weight back onto right leg, bending knee; straighten left knee and flex left foot in Empty Step. As you shift weight, draw both arms inward: bend left elbow and make a right angle with forearm up in a perpendicular; fist the hand, facing fist—palm north. At the same time, fist the right hand and place it under left elbow; both wrists are straight. Right fist-palm faces inward. (Fig. 63)

### Form 20. Brush Knee Twist Step    *Lou Hsi Niu Pu*

Going backward on left side

Shift weight forward onto left foot, bending left knee, and straighten right knee; body is on a slant forward west in Walking Step position. At the same time, bend left fist north and then forward to west, moving left arm to west shoulder high, straightening elbow and opening left hand: palm faces north with fingers to west. Right fist remains under left elbow. (Fig. 64)

Draw left arm closely inward toward body by bending elbow downward, bending wrist so that fingers remain pointing to west with palm north. Right fist is still under left elbow. At the same time shift weight back onto right leg, bending knee, and straighten left knee, flexing foot (Empty Step). (Fig. 65)

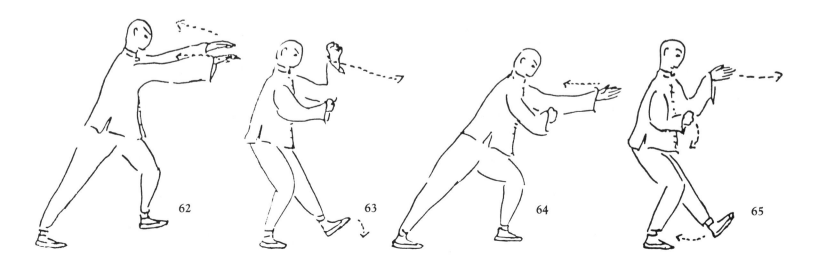

62    63    64    65

Without touching floor, draw left foot with loose ankle close to right foot. At the same time left arm moves outward to level of left shoulder; open right hand gradually and start to move it downward toward right thigh. (Fig. 66)

Weight remains on right leg with its bent knee. Place left foot backward behind body, to east, in the Walking Step Space, and straighten knee. Body slants forward west. As the left leg moves, continue to move left arm forward west in line with left shoulder, turning hand to face west, while right hand finishes its movement at front of right thigh, with palm down and fingers west. (Fig. 67)

Brush Knee Twist Step
Going backward on right side

Shift weight back onto left leg, bending left knee; straighten right knee and flex right foot (Empty Step). Draw left hand inward to center, ten inches from chest, keeping elbow high; palm faces west with fingers pointing north. At the same time, move right hand upward above left wrist, pointing fingers west, with palm south. (Fig. 68)

Without touching floor, draw right foot with loose ankle close to left. Keep weight on left leg. Place right foot behind toward east in the Walking Step Space, straightening knee. At the same time, both arms continue to move: move right arm forward in line with right shoulder, turning palm to west. Circle left arm downward to front of left thigh, with palm down and fingers pointing to west. (Fig. 69)

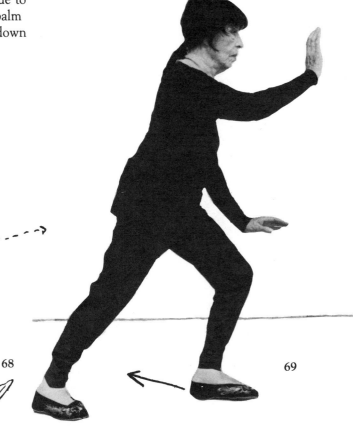

66    67    68    69

Going backward on left side

Shift weight back onto right leg, bending knee; straighten left knee and flex foot (Empty Step). Draw right hand inward to center, ten inches away from chest, keeping elbow high: palm faces west with fingers pointing south. At the same time, move left hand upward above right wrist, pointing fingers west, with palm facing north.

Without touching floor, draw left foot with loose ankle in to right foot. Keep weight on right leg. Place left foot back toward east in the Walking Step Space, straightening knee. Body slants forward west. At the same time, both arms continue to move: move left arm forward west in line with left shoulder, turning palm toward west. Circle right arm downward to front of right thigh, with palm down, and fingers pointing west. (Fig. 67)

**Form 21. Flying Oblique**     *Hsieh Fei Shih*

Keep weight on right leg with its bent knee. Foot, hand, and head move together. Turn toes of right foot to northwest. Turn right palm up, keeping fingers pointing to west. Bend head down, and turn chin toward right shoulder. Do not move arm or shoulders; do not shift weight from right leg. Movements are made in ankle, wrist, and neck. (Fig. 70)

Keep weight on right leg with its bent knee. (1) Turn torso to northwest; right arm will then be at right side of right leg. (2) Bend torso, bending left knee lower; this releases left leg—knee bends, heel rises, keep toes on floor. Right hand is at knee level. (Fig 71) (3) Move left foot inward to right foot and continue to move left leg outward toward southwest, as far as it can go and straighten knee. See arrows for foot movement in Figure 71. Place left foot parallel to right foot. Now both feet point northwest.

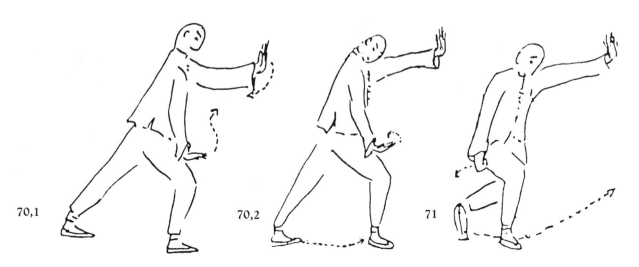

70,1                                    70,2                                    71

64     At the same time continue to circle right hand while left leg goes southwest, with palm up, inward to northeast; fingers point to northeast. (Fig. 72) (4) Shift weight onto left leg, bending left knee and straightening right knee. Torso is forward and faces northwest. Head looks northeast. At the same time, as weight shifts to left leg, turn left palm up with fingers pointing west, and straighten wrist. At the same time, turn right palm down, with fingers pointing northeast. Right arm is parallel to right leg. Look at back of right hand. All these movements finish together. (Fig. 73)

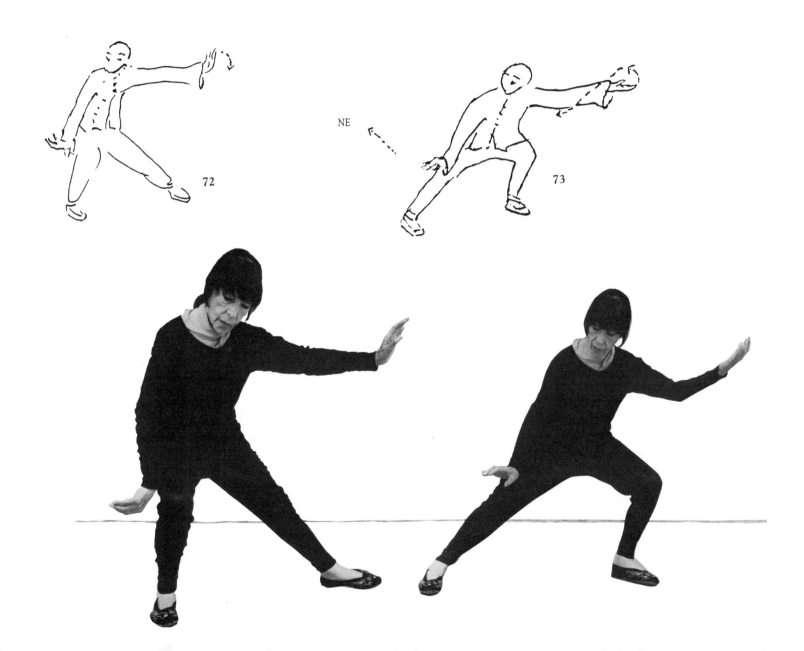

## Form 22. Raise Hands and Step Up   *T'i Shou Shang Shih*

The same as Form 6, Figure 35, 36, 37.

Turn right toes to point north and shift weight onto right leg, bending right knee, and straighten left knee. On this movement straighten torso and turn torso to face north. Then turn toes of left foot to point north. At same time, turn right palm sideways with straight wrist; lift it up northeast shoulder high. Then curve right elbow bringing right hand over to left side shoulder level, palm inward. Move left hand with palm turned toward northeast, toward inner curve of right elbow. Left elbow points downward and right elbow is chest high. (Fig. 74) As arms move, torso bends forward north.

Draw left foot up and place it parallel and apart from right foot, in the basic stance. Both knees are bent equally and torso is curved forward north. At the same time, the arms complete the movements described above: right arm is curved forward shoulder high, and left palm is at inner curve of right elbow. Legs and arms finish together. (See Fig. 36)

Raise body to an upright position, at the same time, straightening knees. Also at the same time, lift curved right arm to a position near forehead, and lower left arm, with palm down, to front of left thigh: wrist is bent and fingers point north. Arms, body, and legs finish together. (See Fig. 37)

Then, as a separate movement, turn the right hand to face palm upward; bending wrist.

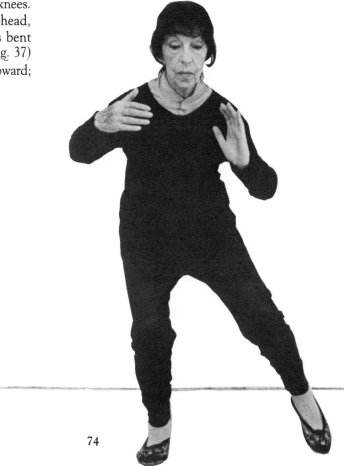

74

### Form 23. White Stork Flaps Its Wings  *Pai Hao Liang Ch'ih*

Same as Form 7, Figures 38, 39, 40, 41, 42

Do not move right arm from its place near forehead for the next sequences.

Bend torso forward down, and, at the same time, move left arm away from thigh so that it is perpendicular to floor, palm facing floor; hand is knee level. (Fig. 38)

Keep arms in same relative positions. Twist torso around to west, keeping body low. Arms move with body. Now left fingers point west. (Fig. 39, 75)

Lift torso up erect, remaining turned west. At the same time bring straight left arm up shoulder high. Left wrist is bent with palm west, and fingers point upward; eyes look at left hand. (Fig. 40)

Turn torso to north. As you do this, bend left elbow and bring left hand to center of forehead, with palm north, so that left fingers point to right fingers; right palm is north. Finger tips of hands are close but do not touch. Hands are a fist length away from forehead. (Fig. 41)

Bend both knees, keeping back straight. At the same time, move both hands: bend wrists and turn hands so that palms face diagonally front-downward: At the same time as hands move, press elbows diagonally forward so that right elbow points northeast and left points northwest, both being at shoulder level. Make this movement with strength and hardness. Feel the tensed contraction in the muscles of upper arms. This contrasts with the light intrinsic movement you have been using up to now. Feel as if you were holding or pressing the upper half of a ball between elbows and hands. Knees and hands move together. (Fig. 42)

### Form 24. Brush Knee Twist Step  *Lou Hsi Niu Pu*

Right side — same as in Form 8, Figures 43, 44

Keeping weight on right leg with its bent knee, shift right heel to the east. This movement turns torso to face west, and at the same time, the weight is released from left leg. Then straighten left knee and flex left foot. As body and legs turn to west, turn right palm inward toward forehead, and turn left palm outward. Then circle left arm outward and downward, and move right arm down while left hand goes under the right hand as right hand circles above left wrist. By this time you are facing west. Both hands are ten inches away from chest: right palm faces south with fingers pointing west. Left wrist is bent, with fingers north and palm west. (Fig. 43)

Moving left leg west, place heel in the Empty Step Space, with straight knee and flexed foot. Then transfer weight onto left leg, bending left knee and straightening right knee. Body slants forward west. As you step west, both arms move: move right arm to west in line with right shoulder, turning palm to face west with fingers pointing upward. At the same time, circle left arm with bent wrist downward, and place left hand in front of left thigh. Palm faces down with fingers pointing west. (Fig. 44)

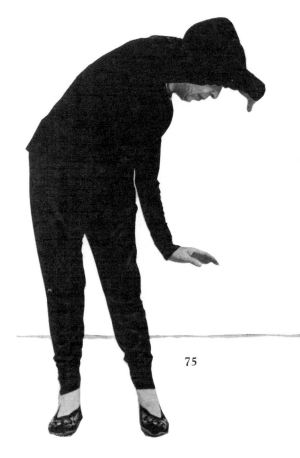

75

**Form 25. Hand Strums the Lute** *Shou U Hui P'i-P'a*

Same as Form 9, Figure 45

Shift weight back onto right leg, bending right knee and, at the same time, straighten left knee and flex foot. As legs move, both arms move: bring right arm inward nine inches from face, keeping right palm facing west with fingers pointing up. Move left hand upward, and place finger tips at right pulse; left palm faces inward toward heart. Arms and legs move at the same time. (Fig. 76)

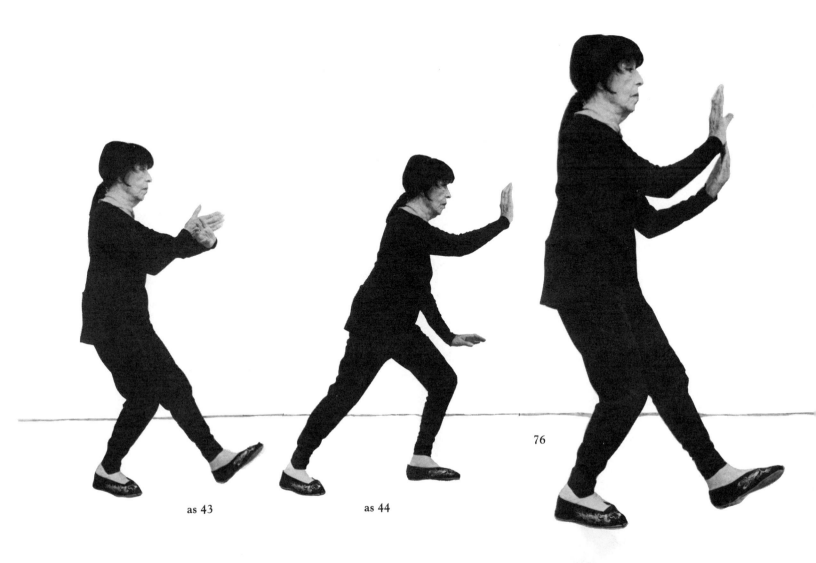

as 43       as 44       76

### Form 26. Needle at the Bottom of the Sea    *Hai Ti Chen*

Draw left foot with loose ankle close to right foot, touching toes by bending right knee more deeply, and lean torso forward on a diagonal. Keep spine straight—do not curve the back. On body and leg movement, move both arms: turning right palm south and left palm north, move right arm diagonally downward, with straight wrist, and gradually straighten right elbow. At the same time, move left palm close along right forearm to right inner elbow: left wrist bends gradually. Right arm is straight; left wrist and elbow are bent. Arms, leg, and body finish together. (Fig. 77)

### Form 27. Fan Through the Back    *Shan T'ung Pei*

Keep weight on right leg. Raise torso and direct it to northwest angle. At same time, lift up both arms, pointing right fingers to northwest angle, at shoulder level; left hand remains at right inner elbow.

   Then place left foot at side of right, with left heel in line with right toes, turning left toes inward to point northwest. Straighten left knee. Right knee is close to left leg. Head looks northwest. (Fig. 78)

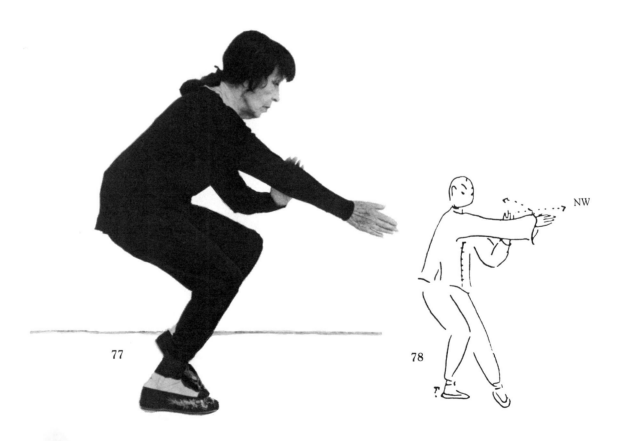

77

78

NW

Shift weight onto left leg, bending left knee and straightening right knee. At the same time, begin to move both arms: slide (do not touch) left fingers along right forearm toward northwest and draw right arm to right side. Left finger tips are at right palm when left knee is bent and right knee is straight. Keep left elbow down. Right elbow is in line with right hand. (Fig. 79)

Keeping weight on bent left leg, move right heel slightly inward, making foot parallel to left foot. Then turn right toes outward to point northeast, bending right knee to equal left knee bend. You are now seated evenly on both legs, facing northeast. As you move right heel and toes, continue to move both arms: move left arm, which is shoulder high, to northwest with palm facing northwest and fingers up. At the same time, move bent right arm, elbow leading, toward the right until hand is opposite right shoulder and elbow is in line with right shoulder toward southeast. Move right hand upward toward right ear and place near the neck and bend wrist with palm up. Head is turned to left hand, eyes look at back of left hand. (Fig. 80)

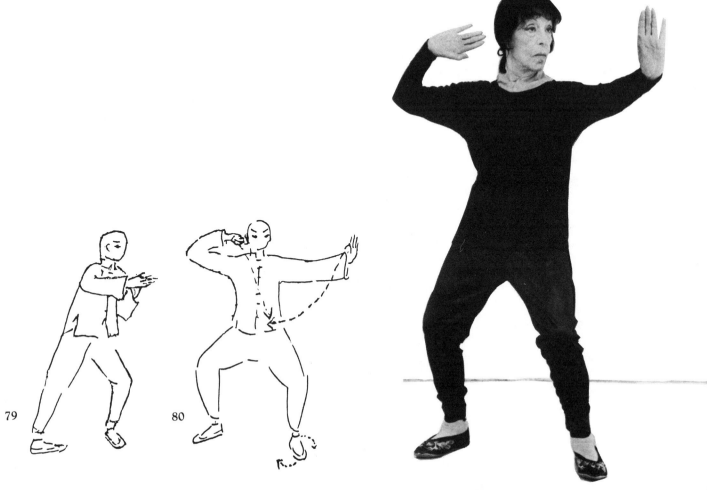

79        80

### Form 28. Turn Body—Throw Fist   *Fan Shen P'ieh Shen Ch'ui*

Keeping weight on left leg with bent knee, move left toes slightly inward to northeast; then move left heel outward to west, and on this heel movement straighten right knee. Keep right foot on floor. As left toes and heel move, upper torso is shifted to face northeast; head is now looking north. While you move left toes and heel, both arms move: circle left arm downward, finger tips inward, make hand into a fist and place it near left hip-bone, with fist-palm facing down. Circle right arm, making hand into a fist, downward and inward toward left hip, finger tips inward. Place right fist above left, with fist-palms down. Both fists arrive in position at the same time, with movement of left heel. When fists meet, pull shoulders forward, moving elbows forward; left elbow points north and right elbow points east. Use a hard force, similar to "pressing the ball," Form 7. (Fig. 81)

Move right toes to point east, shifting weight onto right leg, bending right knee, and straightening left knee. Body slants forward east. At the same time, both arms move: move right fist up to east, chest high, with fist-palm facing east; wrist is bent. Move left fist, staying close behind right fist, gradually opening hand and spreading fingers wide apart behind right. Left palm faces right fist, with left fingers pointing upward. Both wrists are bent; both elbows are low. (Fig. 82)

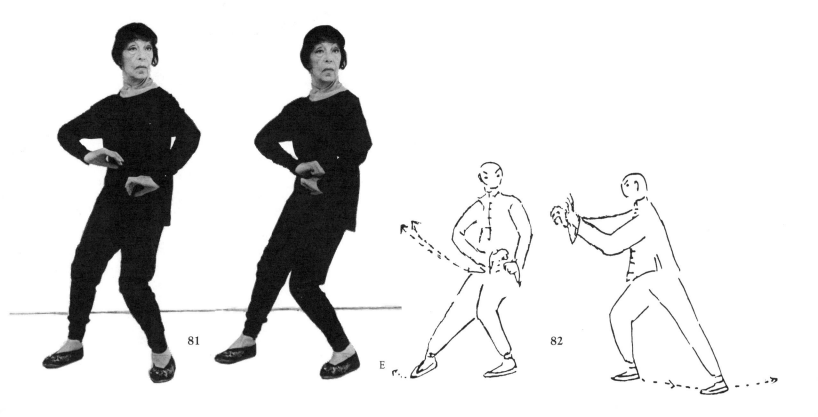

81
E
82

## Form 29. Step Up, Parry, and Punch    *Chin Pu Pan Lan Ch'ui*

Shift weight back onto left leg, bending knee, straightening right leg, and flexing foot. At the same time, both hands move: turn left palm to face south, chest high, and gradually place fingers together; turn right fist to face left, palm. Draw right fist toward right hip, turning fist-palm upward, elbow moving back to point west. At the same time as right arm is drawing back, place left hand forward at height of left shoulder, with palm south. Draw right foot with loose ankle back to left foot (not touching floor).

Do not move left arm. At same time, step right foot backward in Walking Step Space; place weight on right leg, bending right knee, straightening left knee, and flexing foot. On this last shifting of weight onto right leg, draw right fist to right hip, with elbow back to point west. Fist-palm faces upward; left arm remains forward east, in line with left shoulder. (Fig. 83)

Shift weight forward onto left leg, bending its knee, and straighten right knee. Body slants forward east. At the same time, both arms move: bring right fist forward east, shoulder high, with fist-palm facing north, and move left palm to right inner elbow, bending left elbow and wrist. (Fig. 84)

## Form 30. Grasping the Bird's Tail    *Lan Ch'üeh Wei*

Similar to Forms 2, 3, 4, Figures 25, 26, 27, 28, 29.

Shift weight back onto right leg, bending right knee, straightening left knee, and flexing foot. At the same time, move left fingers to right pulse and open right hand with fingers pointing east in Grasping Bird's Tail Form, at chest level (Fig. 25 for arms).

Keep the relationship of hands the same: move both arms inward toward the body at chest level, with both elbows bent downward and slightly out until right wrist is nine inches in front of chest. (Fig. 25)

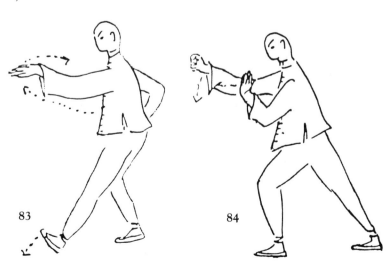

83        84

Turn right palm up and left palm down. As you move hands, angle left hand so that it is at right angles to right wrist and left elbow points north. At same time as hands turn, shift weight forward onto left leg, bending left knee and straightening right knee; body is on a diagonal forward to east. Then draw right foot with loose ankle close to left foot. Form 2 does not contain this step.

Place right heel forward east in the Empty Step Space, bending right knee and straightening left knee. From this point on, this pattern is like Forms 4 and 4. Body slants forward. At the same time as you step forward, stretch right arm to northeast, straightening right elbow. Keep left fingers at right wrist. (Fig. 27)

Circle both arms horizontally shoulder high, going from northeast to east, to southeast. When arms reach southeast bend right elbow downward, bending right wrist so that palm faces upward. Left fingers stay at right pulse. Left arm is adjusted to movement of right arm. (Fig. 28)

As you are circling, when arms move from southeast, shift weight back onto left leg, bending left knee, and straighten right knee, flexing foot. Turn right fingers to southeast. (Fig. 28)

Pivoting on right heel, turn right toes to northeast. At the same time, raise right arm, with palm leading upward, arcing head high. Circle it over and down toward northeast, straightening arm as you do so, and stop in position when right wrist is slightly above shoulder height. At same time, place toes on floor.

As you are approaching this last position with right arm, bend right knee, placing weight on right leg, and straighten left knee. Then bend right wrist and lower hand, making fingers point downward, and place all fingers over thumb in Grasping position: right arm remains in place while hand moves. Left fingers remain near right pulse; left palm faces your face. Left wrist is straight; arm is curved. (Fig. 29; 85)

### Form 31. The Single Whip     *Tan Pien*
Same as Form 5, Figures 30, 31, 32

Hold weight firmly on right leg with its bent knee. Draw left foot with loose ankle close to right without touching floor. Then move left leg backward to southwest diagonal in the Walking Step Space. Straighten left knee and place foot parallel to right foot. Weight is on right bent leg and body is on diagonal slant toward northeast. As left leg moves, move left arm, with palm toward face, in a downward curve in toward body, chest high. Left palm is toward the face; arm is curved. Right arm does not move. (Fig. 30)

Continue moving left arm up and outward toward northwest, and then pivoting on left heel, turn toes to point northwest. Place weight on left leg and bend knee to equal bend of right knee. Now your weight is even on both legs. Body is turned northwest. As left foot moves, turn left palm to face northwest. Now both arms are at same level, with wrists slightly higher than shoulder level. Right arm is extended toward northeast, left arm is extended northwest, and left palm faces northwest. (Fig. 31)

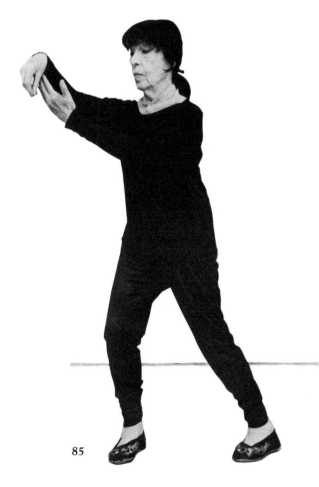

85

Same as Form 5

   Look at left palm. Keep looking at it as hand moves to northwest. Turn head from right to left side, but do *not* bend head downward when eyes look downward. The top of head is kept level as head moves from right to left side. On last movement of left hand to northwest position, look at back of left hand. Left arm, left leg, eyes, and torso move together. (Fig. 86)

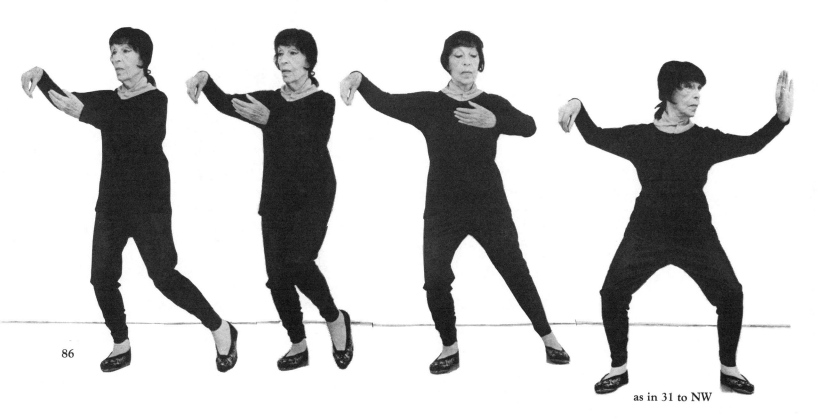

86

**as in 31 to NW**

## Form 32. Cloud Arms    *Yŭn Shou*

Do not move right arm. Turn left toes inward to north and then move left heel outward to make left foot parallel with right foot. With movements of left foot, shift weight onto right leg and straighten left knee; body slants to northeast. At the same time as you move left foot and shift weight, circle left arm downward and then inward to body, abdomen high. Gradually straightening wrist, move left arm upward toward right wrist. Place left fingers near right pulse, with palm inward facing you. As left arm moves, raise right hand slowly upward, opening hand to face palm northeast. Left foot, left arm, and right hand all move together. (Fig. 87)

(1) Shift weight back onto left leg, bending left knee and straightening right knee. Feel as if you were sitting on left leg. Torso is erect; back is straight. As weight shifts, move both arms at the same time. (2) Turn torso north. Looking at left palm, move left arm, with palm at eye level, to within twelve inches of face. Keep eyes fixed on palm. At the same time, circle right arm outward to right side, and then downward, with bent wrist and palm facing down. (Fig. 88) (3) Keeping weight on left leg, turn right toes inward to point northwest. (4) Turn left toes outward to point northwest. As feet move, torso moves to face northwest. At the same time, both arms move: continue to move left arm, face high, to left side with eyes looking at palm. Continue to move right arm in its circle, from downward to inward, abdomen high in front of body, gradually straightening wrist. (Fig. 89)

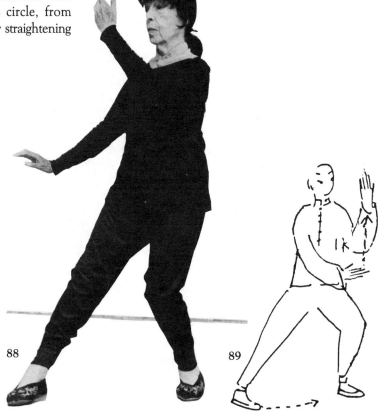

87          88          89

(5) Keeping weight on left leg, place right foot parallel and apart from left in your basic stance: both toes point northwest, both knees are evenly bent, and back is straight. Torso faces nortwest. Both arms continue to move: turn left palm to face northwest, at eye level, while you move right fingers up to left pulse, turning right palm toward your face. Look at right palm. Both elbows point downward. (Fig. 90) (6) Turn torso toward right to face north and move right arm to right side, with palm at eye level, twelve inches away from face. At the same time move left arm straight out to west with palm west. Eyes are looking at right palm. (7) Then turn right toes to northeast, placing weight on right leg with its bent knee. At same time, lower left arm downward to within eight inches of thigh. Torso with right arm still has turned northeast. (8) Turn left knee inward, touching left toes to floor, with loose ankle, thus taking weight off left foot. At the same time both arms move: left moves across body, abdomen high in an arc; right elbow begins to unbend with hand slowly turning, moving toward the northeast. (Fig. 91) (9) As the left hand goes up toward the right side, place left leg diagonally backward to southwest, in the Walking Step Space. Straighten left knee. Weight is on right leg. Body slants to northeast. On this last movement, turn right palm out to face northeast straightening elbow and place left fingers at right pulse with palm toward face. At this moment eyes look far away toward the northeast. Left hand, right hand, left leg movement, and shifting eye gaze are all made at the same time. (Fig. 87)

Repeat Cloud Arms—Figures 88, 89, 90, 91, and 87—again in exactly the same way. Do not omit this repeat.

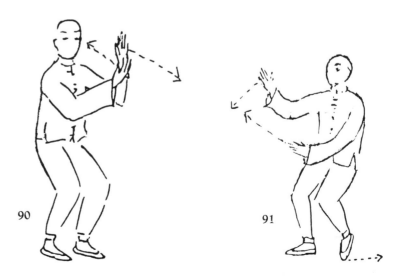

90                    91

### Form 33. The Single Whip    *Tan Pien*

Same as Form 5, Figures 30, 31, 32

Continue this from the repeat of Form 32. Bend right wrist downward and place fingers in Grasping position.

Then move left arm downward and in toward the body, chest high; then upward to northwest. (Fig. 30)

Turn left palm to face northwest and at the same time turn left toes to point northwest; bend left knee even with right knee. Back is straight.

As left arm moves, look at left palm as it moves downward and upward. Move head from right to left side. Look at back of left hand on its last movement. Torso faces northwest. (Fig. 92)

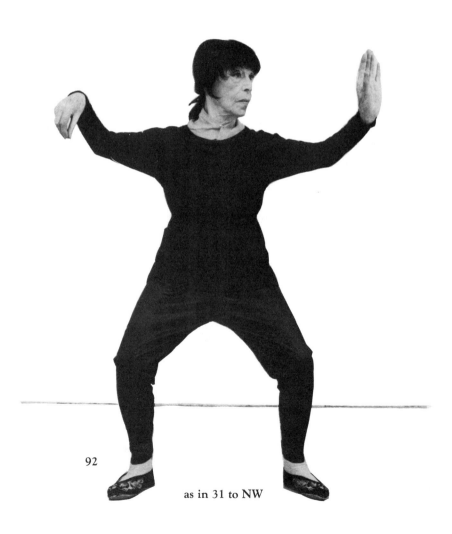

92

as in 31 to NW

**Form 34. On Right—High Pat the Horse**    *Kao T'an Ma*

Keeping weight on right leg, move right toes inward slightly; then move right heel outward to east, and straighten left knee, keeping left foot on floor. This movement on right foot turns torso to west. At the same time as you move right foot, bend right elbow downward and raise right hand upward, opening hand. Then bring hand inward toward right shoulder with palm south. Left palm now faces north. (Fig. 93)

Weight remains on right leg with its bent knee. Draw left foot with loose ankle and place it close to right foot; touch toes (i.e. ball of foot, not tip-toes) to floor. Back is straight. At the same time, both arms move: move left palm upward, draw left arm downward, left elbow goes to left side at hip height. Palm is up with straight wrist. Move right arm upward west with palm turned to south; keep elbow high so that hand is at face level. Right elbow is bent almost at a right angle. Left palm is in the same vertical plane as right elbow. Arms are separated by width of body. (Fig. 94)

**Form 35. On Left—Open Body**    *Tso P'i Shen*

Place left heel forward west in the Empty Step Space; then transfer weight onto left leg, bending left knee and straightening right knee. Body is on a slant toward west. At the same time, both arms move: turn both palms down and move both hands downward toward the center, abdomen high. Right hand goes above the left hand; wrists are crossed; right fingers point southwest; left fingers point northwest. Arms are straight, with wrists centered, abdomen high. (Fig. 95)

Do not move body, legs, or head for next sequence.

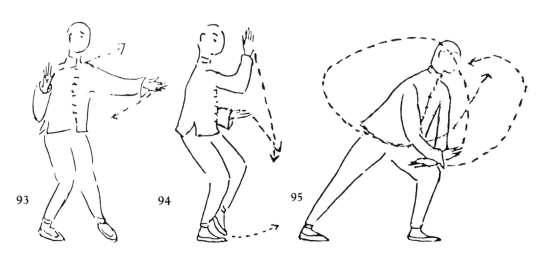

93    94    95

Both arms move together. Bend both elbows slightly. Circle left arm outward to south, then upward to shoulder level, turning palm to face west with fingers pointing south. Elbow is straight. Then bend left elbow at shoulder level, and bring left hand, making a fist of it, to left ear: wrist is straight and fist-palm faces west. At the same time, right arm moves: bring right arm upward as high as forehead with palm up; then move it outward, straightened, toward north with palm north and fingers up; then turning palm east, straightening wrist, bring arms down across body at abdomen, height; then bend elbow and bring hand up to left side: make a fist of right hand and place it in front of left fist. Wrist-pulses face each other, without touching. Right elbow, in horizontal plane with left elbow, points west. Both wrists side-bend up so that knuckles point upward. (Fig. 96)

Then turn head to look north. Do not tilt head. (Fig. 96)

Now turn right fist-palm to face west. Then open both hands spreading fingers very wide apart. Direct fingers to point upward; do not move elbows. Legs and torso and head have remained still. (Fig. 97)

**Form 36. Raise Right Leg**     *T'i Yu Chiao*

Shift weight onto left leg. Draw right foot with loose ankle close to left foot and stand, straightening left knee. Then raise right leg up toward northwest angle. Leg is straight; foot is turned inward, with toes leading (see page 30). At the same time, move both arms: move right arm to shoulder level, toward northwest, with palm facing southwest, straight wrist. Move left arm curved outward toward southeast: palm faces southeast and is at head level, wrist is bent and fingers point upward. (Fig. 98) When arms move, place fingers together, normally.

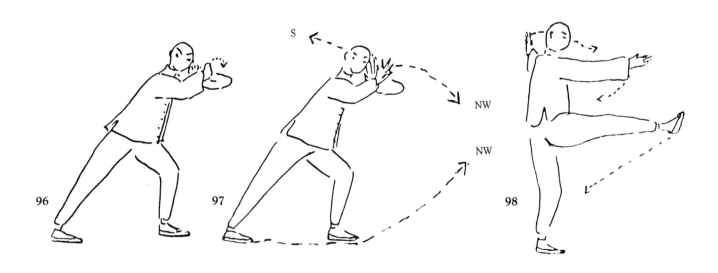

S

NW

NW

96          97          98

## Form 37. On Left—High Pat the Horse    *Kao T'an Ma'*

Bend right leg raising knee slightly. Then bring foot with loose ankle close to left knee. At the same time, bend left elbow down, hand near shoulder. Right arm does not move. (Fig. 99)

Bending left knee, place right toes on floor lightly. At the same time, both arms move into position: turn right palm upward and left palm north; then move left arm toward west with palm north, keeping left elbow high so that hand is at face level. Left elbow is bent almost at a right angle. Right elbow goes near right hip; right palm is in plane of left elbow, and arms are separated by width of body. (Fig. 100)

## Form 38. On Right—Open Body    *Yu P'i Shen*

Reverse of Figures 95, 96, 97

Place right heel forward west in the Empty Step space; then transfer weight onto right leg, bending knee and straightening left knee. Body is on a slant forward west. At the same time, both arms move: turn both palms down and move both hands downward toward the center, abdomen high. Left hand goes above right hand, wrists are crossed, left fingers point northwest, and right fingers point southwest. Arms are straight, hands centered. (Reverse of Figure 95)

Do not move body, legs, or head for next sequence.

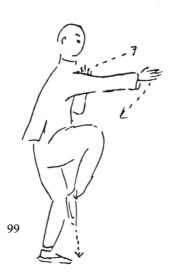

99

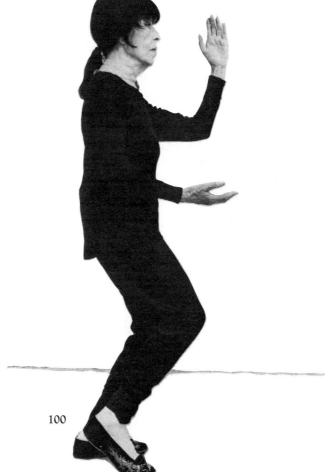

100

Both arms move together. Bend both elbows slightly; circle right arm outward to north, then upward to shoulder level, straightening elbows, turning palm to face west with fingers pointing north. Then bend right elbow at shoulder level and bring hand, closing it to a fist, to right ear. Wrist is straight and fist-palm faces west. At the same time, left arm moves: bring left arm upward as high as forehead with palm up; then move it outward toward south, with straight elbow, with palm south and fingers upward; then downward, turning palm east and straightening wrist across body; then up, bending elbow, over toward right side making a fist of left hand and bringing it in front of right fist. Wrist-pulses face each other and do not touch. Left elbow, in horizontal plane with right elbow, points west. Both wrists side-bend up so that knuckles point upward. (Reverse of Figure 96)

Then turn head to look south. Do not tilt head. (Reverse of Figure 96)

Now turn left fist-palm to face west. Open both hands, spreading fingers very wide apart from each other. Direct fingers to point to ceiling; do not move elbows. Legs and torso and head have remained still. (Fig. 97)

### Form 39. Raise Left Leg    *T'i Tso Chiao*

Shift weight onto right leg. Draw left foot with loose ankle, close to right foot, not touching floor. Stand, straightening right knee. Then raise left leg up toward southwest angle. Leg is straight; foot is turned inward, with toes leading (see page 30). At the same time, both arms move: move left arm at shoulder level toward the southwest, palm facing northwest, with wrist straight. Move right arm curved outward toward northeast: palm faces northeast and is above shoulder level; wrist is bent, and fingers point upward. (Fig. 101) When arms move, place fingers together, normally.

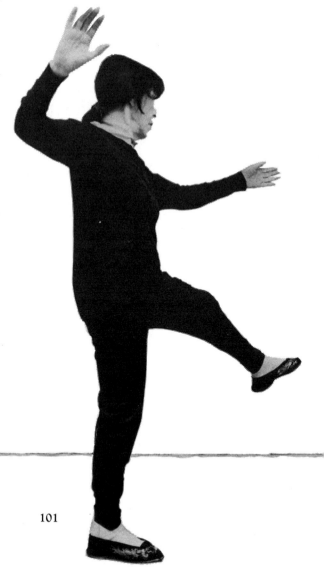

101

## Form 40. Pivot Body on Heel—Raise Leg     *Chuan Shen Teng Chiao*

Bend left knee, raising it slightly. Move leg so that knee points west, and place left foot with loose ankle close to right knee: left foot is turned inward (see page 30). At the same time, both arms move: make a fist of right hand and bring it near right ear with elbow at shoulder level, pointing north. Make fist of left hand and bring it in front of right wrist, with pulses facing each other. Elbow is same height as right elbow. Head does not move: it faces south; weight is on right leg. (Fig. 102)

Keep arms and head in position. Quickly pivot on right heel, turning body to face south by placing right toes to point directly south. Head looks east now. Fists remain near right ear; right elbow now points west. (Fig. 103)

Then turn left fist outward to face south.

Now open both hands and spread fingers wide apart, fingers pointing upward.

Raise left leg directly to east and flex foot (see page 30). At the same time, both arms move: move right arm to west, so that hand with wrist bent is at head level: palm is west and fingers point up. Move left arm to east shoulder high: palm faces south with fingers east, and wrist is straight. (Fig. 104) When arms move, place fingers together, normally.

## Form 41. Brush Knee and Twist Step     *Lou Hsi Niu Pu*

Draw left leg inward to body, keeping knee high, and place foot with loose ankle near right knee. Bend more deeply on right knee and turn torso to face east. Straightening left knee, place left heel on floor to east in direct line with right heel: weight is on right leg with its bent knee. At the same time, right arm moves bending right elbow downward; draw right hand inward toward right shoulder. As torso shifts to face east, palm also faces east. Keep left arm with palm south in place, not moving. (Fig. 105)

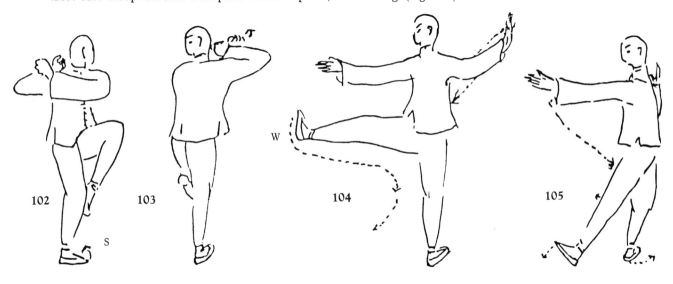

102   103   104   105

82      Shift weight onto left leg, bending its knee and straightening right knee. Body is on a slant toward east. At the same time, both arms continue their movements: bring right arm forward east in line with right shoulder: palm faces east and wrist is bent. Move left arm downward to left side of left thigh, with wrist straight and palm facing thigh. Turn the heel of right foot to west as you finish arm movements. Now feet are parallel and are in the Walking Step position. (Fig. 106)

### Form 42. Plant Leg and Punch Step    *Chin Pu Tsai Ch'ui*

Draw right leg with loose ankle close to left foot, not touching floor. Left knee is bent; weight is on left leg. Both arms move at the same time as right leg moves; circle right arm inward toward center: fingers point north and palm faces east. Move left hand up over right wrist, with fingers pointing to east.

Continue moving arms: circle right hand under left; make a fist of it, turning fist-palm upward. Draw fist toward right hip, with elbow pointing to west, and begin to move left hand, a short distance, with palm south, to east, in line with left shoulder. (Fig. 107)

Step forward east *quickly* on right foot. (Fig 108)

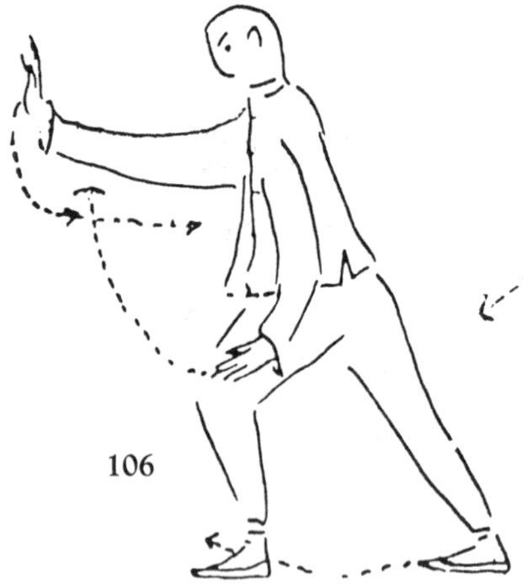

106 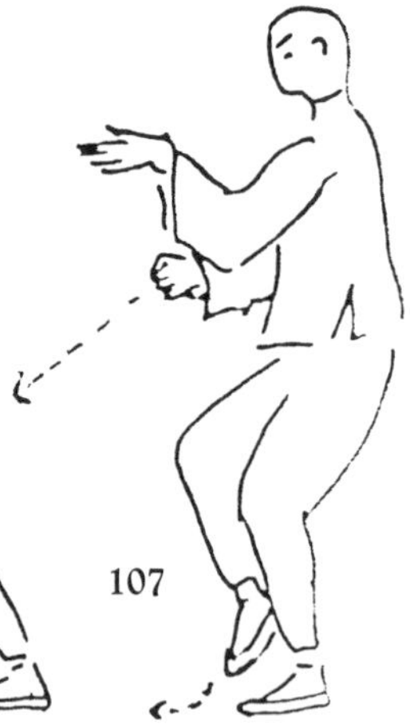              107 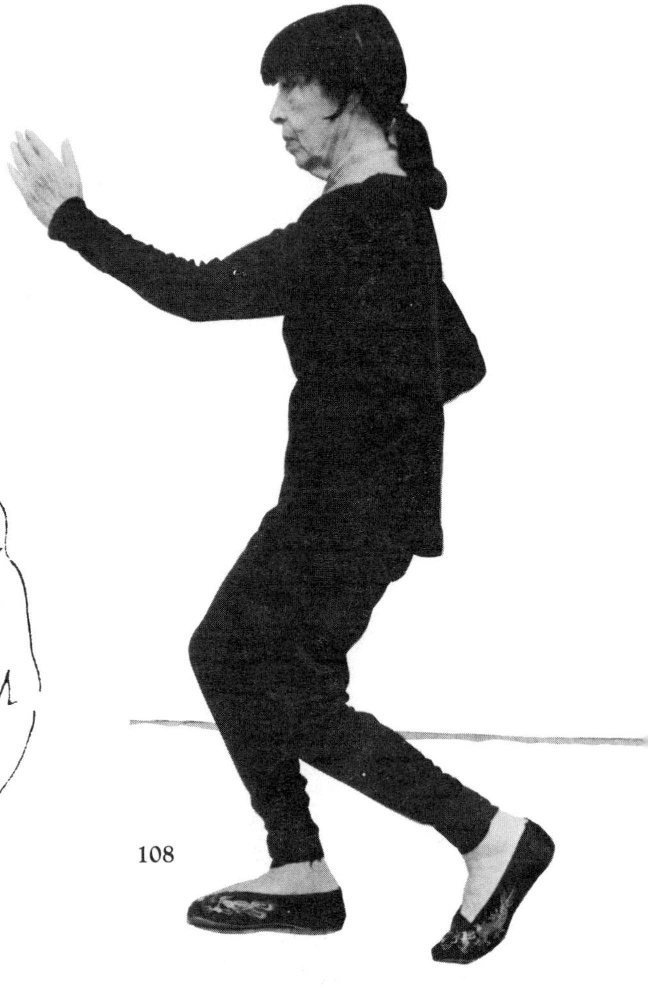              108

Then *quickly* step forward east on left foot, bending its knee and straightening right knee. Weight is forward on left: body slants a diagonal and bends downward, with contracted pelvis. This rhythm is extremely quick—like a flash, moving with a quick step from right to left foot. (Fig. 109)

As you step quickly forward on right leg, both arms also move quickly: pull right fist to right hip and push left arm outward toward east (similar to the gesture of stretching a bow open to shoot an arrow).

Then as you step quickly onto left foot, punch right fist toward east, diagonally downward. At the same time, move left palm to inner right elbow, bending wrist with fingers upward; elbow is bent. This punch is done with hard force. Keep heel of right foot on floor. *Do not move head.* (Fig. 109)

### Form 43. Turn Body—Throw Fist    *Fan Shen P'ien Shen Ch'ui*

Keeping weight on left leg, raise torso to an upright position. At the same time, both arms move: bring left palm up to face right shoulder; bend right elbow, and bring forearm up to cross left forearm, so that right fist-palm faces left shoulder. Both elbows point outward; right arm is on the outer side of this cross. (Fig. 110)

While you are moving torso and both arms into position, start the Toe-Heel-Heel Step (page 32). Feet move as hands are moving together; hands meet when body is southwest. Turn toes of left foot inward to point south. Then turn right heel inward making feet parallel, with weight remaining on left leg: now body faces south. Then turn left heel outward to east; weight is still on left. Now torso faces southwest. Then raise right toes off floor, with right heel touching floor lightly. Now body faces west. (Fig. 111)

While you are raising right toes off floor in Empty Step and turning to face west, both hands move: turn hands to face west; keeping them center, left palm is behind right fist; spread left fingers wide apart. (Fig. 111)

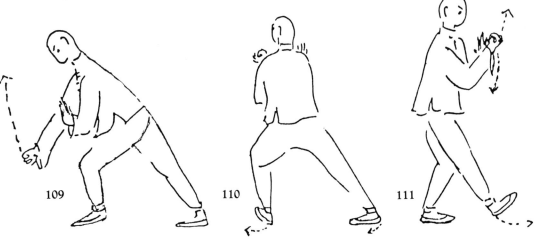

109    110    111

## Form 44. On Right—High Pat the Horse    *Kao T'an Ma*

Same as Form 34, Figure 94

Place right heel forward in the Empty Step Space; transfer weight onto right leg, bending its knee and straightening left knee. At the same time, move left hand, closing fingers, to face right fist which turns to face left hand palm. Place weight on right leg with its bent knee, and draw left toes with loose ankle close to right foot, touching floor. At the same time, turning left palm up, move left arm downward and place elbow near left hip. Move right arm upward and out with palm to south: right elbow and left palm are at same vertical plane. Arms are separated by the width of body. (Fig. 94)

## Form 45. On Left—Open Body    *Tso P'i Shen*

Same as Form 35. Figures 95, 96, 97

Place left heel forward west in the Empty Step Space; then transfer weight onto left leg, bending knee and straightening right knee. Body is on a slant toward west. At the same time, both arms move: turn both palms down and move both hands downward toward the center, abdomen-high. Right hand goes above left hand; wrists are crossed; right fingers point southwest; left fingers point northwest. Both arms are straight and centered. (Fig. 95)

Do not move body, legs, or head for the next sequence.

Both arms move together, bend both elbows slightly. Circle left arm toward south, then up to shoulder level, turning palm to face west, with fingers pointing south. Elbow is straight. Then bend left elbow at shoulder level and bring left hand, closing to a fist, to left ear; wrist is straight and fist-palm faces west. At the same time, right arm moves: bring right arm upward with palm facing up, as high as forehead; then move it outward, straightened, toward north with palm north and fingers up, then downward, turning palm to east straightening wrist. Bring arm downward across body at abdomen height. Then bend elbow and bring hand up to left ear, making a fist of right hand in front of left fist. Wrist-pulses face each other without touching. Right elbow is in horizontal plane with left elbow and points west. Both wrists side-bend up so that knuckles point upward. (Fig. 96)

Turn head to look north. Do not tilt head. (Fig. 96) Turn right fist-palm to face west. Then open both hands, spreading fingers very wide apart. Direct fingers to point upward. Do not move elbows. Legs and torso and head have remained still. (Fig. 97)

**Form 46. Raise Right Leg**     *T'i Yu Chiao*

Same as Form 38, Figure 98

Shift weight onto left leg. Draw right foot with loose ankle close to left foot. Stand and straighten left knee. Then raise right leg toward northwest angle. Leg is straight; foot is turned inward with toes leading. At the same time, both arms move: move right arm, at shoulder level, toward northwest so that palm faces southwest with straight wrist. Move left arm curved outward toward southeast: palm faces southeast and is at head level; wrist is bent and fingers point northwest. (Fig. 98) When arms move, place fingers together, normally.

**Form 47. Retreat Step—Beat the Tiger**     *T'ui Pu Ta Hu*

Weight is on left leg. Bend right knee and bring right foot with loose ankle inward toward left knee. At the same time, left arm moves, bend left elbow downward and turn palm to face northwest, moving hand to left shoulder. (Fig. 112)

Bend left knee, lowering body, and place right foot diagonally back toward southeast, straightening right knee: place right foot so that toes point north. Weight remains on left leg with its bent knee. Body is on a slant diagonally toward the northwest; left toes are pointing west. At the same time as right leg moves, move both arms: move left arm facing palm down toward northwest, finger tips leading, in line with left shoulder. Pulling torso to the right, turn right palm to face up; elbows and wrists are straight. Fingers of both hands point northwest. Head looks northwest. (Fig. 113)

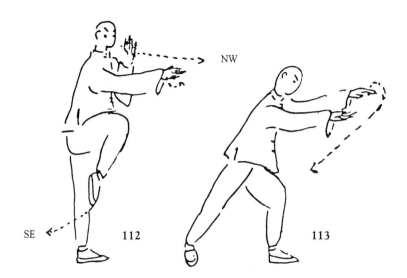

NW

SE

112

113

86    Shift weight back onto right, bending right knee and straighten left knee, and flexing left foot which is therefore angled upward toward west. As you sit back and shift weight onto right leg, bend torso forward and downward over left leg; torso now faces northwest. Move both arms at the same time as legs and torso move: turn left palm up and turn right palm down; place right fingers at left pulse, angling right hand so that it is at right angles to left arm. Right elbow is curved outward. Left arm is straight and parallel to left leg. Legs, torso, and arms move together. (Fig. 114)

Keeping body low, move right hand in a small horizontal circle over left hand, turning left palm to face floor and gradually making hands into fists. Finish right circle movement so that fists are shoulder width apart; both arms are vertical to shoulders. In the meantime, left leg moves: keeping weight on right leg with its bent knee, move left leg diagonally toward southeast, straightening knee, and place left foot with toes pointing southwest. Both fists get into place as left foot arrives in its place. Body is bent forward over right bent leg and faces west. Do not drop head. (Fig. 115)

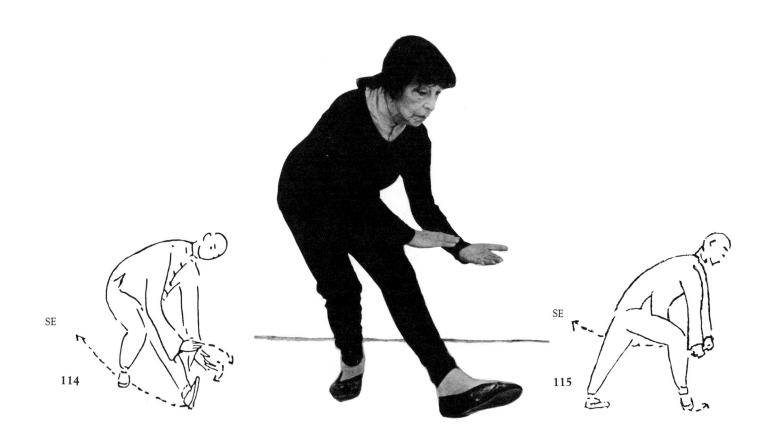

SE    114

SE    115

Swing both arms and torso from right side to left side, and bending left knee, shift weight onto left leg. Turn right toes inward and straighten right knee. Now fists are at knee level at left side, and weight is on left leg. Continue to move torso to twist to left side of waist, moving torso to southeast. (Fig. 116)

Shifting weight from right leg, begin to straighten left knee, lifting torso erect; at same time raise both arms, parallel, up to shoulder height, shoulder width apart. As the left leg straightens, release right leg by raising heel off floor, bending knee; then put right toes near left foot. All these movements are simultaneous. (Fig. 117) Then turn torso to south, arms parallel and shoulder height. (Fig. 118).

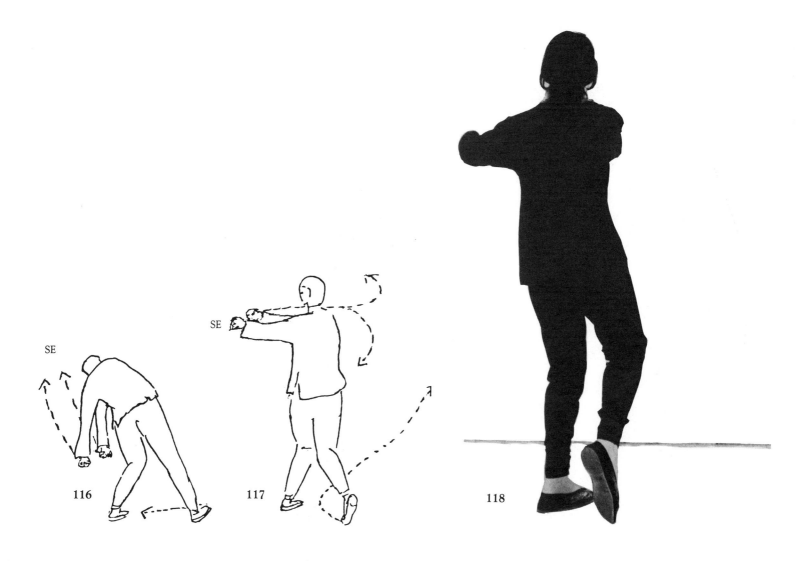

116    117    118

88 Continue west, moving both arms: left arm curves inward toward forehead, right inward toward waist. (Fig. 119) When torso is west, lift right leg forward up with knee *kept* bent so that lower leg is angled out; flex foot. At the finish of leg movement, torso is bent slightly forward; left hand reaches forehead with fist-palm turned out; right fist-palm faces inward, with right elbow touching right knee. (Fig. 120)

### Form 48. Open—Extend Right Leg     *Yu Fen Chiao*

Extend right leg to northwest angle, straightening knee and keeping foot flexed. At the same time, move right arm, opening fist, palm down, above right leg and touch toes with fingers; left arm, with palm to southeast, moves to southeast: fingers are up and wrist is bent. Torso does not move. (Fig. 121)

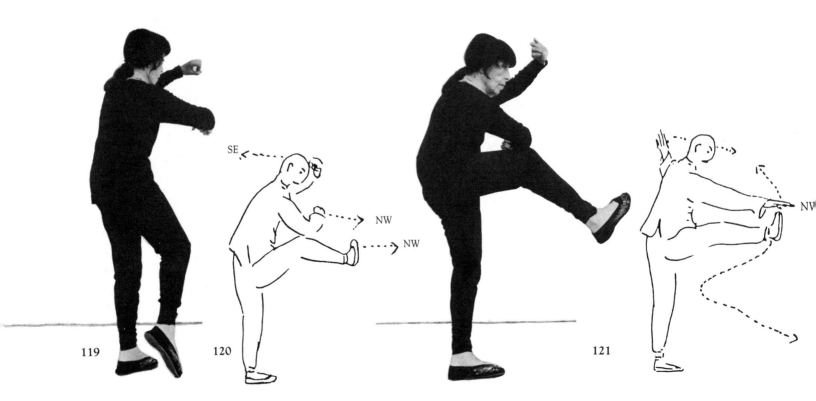

119        120        121

**Form 49. Strike Ears with Fists**     *Shuang Feng Kuan Erh*

Bend right knee and bring right foot with loose ankle close to left knee. Bending left knee, place right heel forward west in the Empty Step Space; then transfer weight onto right leg, bending its knee and straighten left knee: body slants forward to west. At the same time, move left arm inward toward left shoulder, palm facing west; right arm does not move. Place hands near forehead, finger tips pointing to each other; palms face west. When legs move to walking stance, elbows point outward, right to north and left to south. Hands are a fist-length away from forehead. (Fig. 122)

Do not move legs, torso, or head. Move both arms downward vertically, in front of body: palms face floor, wrists are bent, and arms are curved, centered to abdomen. Move arms simultaneously in opposite directions, keeping fingers pointing inward and wrists bent. Move right arm outward to north, and move left outward to south, hip-distance apart, abdomen level, then up to shoulder level. Bending elbows, turn palms west, and bring hands up to center of forehead, making fists of them. Arms have described a vertically curved circle. Fists are a fist-length away from forehead. (Fig. 122, except that hands are now fisted.)

**Form 50. Turn Body—Open Body**     *Fan Shen Yu P'i Shen*

Weight is on right leg with bent knee. Turn toes of right foot to point north, and twist torso to face northwest. Pull right elbow to right side, east, in line with right shoulder; place right fist near right ear. With movement of right arm, move left arm over to right side and place left wrist in front of right wrist. Fist-palms face each other. Head remains looking west. Right toes, torso, and arms move and finish at the same time. (Fig. 123)

Turn left fist-palm to face north. Then open hands, spreading fingers very wide apart, and direct fingers to point upward.

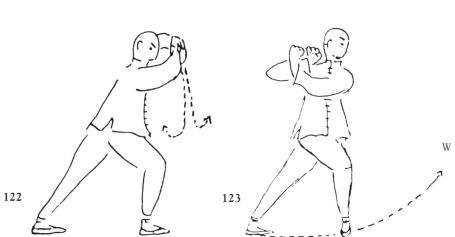

122

123

W

**Form 51. Raise the Left Leg**     *T'i Tso Chiao*

Draw left foot with loose ankle to right foot. Torso faces north, legs are close. Then raise left leg directly to west with straightened knee and flexed foot. On leg movement, separate arms: move left arm to west shoulder high, with wrist straight and palm north. Move right arm to east, bending wrist and turning palm to face east with fingers pointing upward. (Fig. 124) When arms move, place fingers together, normally.

**Form 52. Turn the Body—Open**     *Fan Shen Tso P'i Shen*

Swing left leg around right leg *quickly* pivoting on ball of right foot, and turn to face south. Place left foot with out-turned toes, in front of—therefore to the south of—right foot. All this is done quickly. Adjust weight firmly on left foot. Move left toes to point south: left knee is straight, and right knee is bent, with right heel *off* ground, toes touching floor. As you make this quick turn, bend left elbow shoulder high, make a fist of left hand, and bring it to left ear; at the same time, right elbow will bend while turning. Make a right fist, and place right wrist in front of left wrist. As you make the quick turn and as you cross your wrists, head turns to look west. All movements with legs, head, and arms are done as quickly as possible. (Fig. 125)

In basic tempo again turn right fist-palms to face south. Open hands, spreading fingers very wide apart; direct fingers to point upward. While you are moving hands, fix weight firmly on left leg so that right leg is free to move.

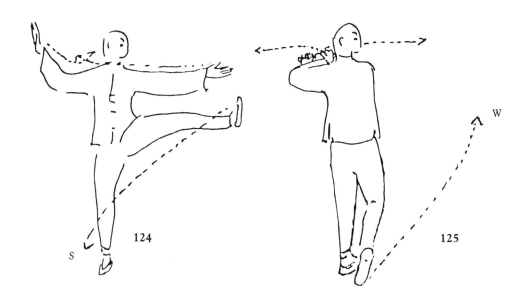

124

125

S

W

**Form 53. Raise the Right Leg**    *T'i Yu Chiao*

Raise right leg directly to west with straightened knee and flexed foot. With this leg movement, separate arms: move right arm to west shoulder high, with wrist straight and palm south; move left arm to east, bending wrist and turning palm to east with fingers pointing upward. (Fig. 126) When arms move, place fingers together, normally.

**Form 54. Step Up, Parry, and Punch**    *Chin Pu Pan Lan Ch'ui*

Similar to Form 12, Figures 48, 49

Bend right knee and bring right foot with loose ankle near left knee. At the same time, bend left elbow downward and bring hand to shoulder with palm south. Right arm does not move. (Fig. 127)

With weight on left leg, bend knee, place right heel forward west in the Empty Step Space; then transfer weight onto right leg, bending its knee, and straightening left knee. At the same time, move left heel outward to make foot parallel to right foot. As heel moves, move left arm gradually forward west in line with left shoulder, with palm facing north. Right arm does not move. (Fig. 128)

Move left foot with loose ankle close to right foot. Then place heel forward west in the Empty Step Space, and transfer weight onto left leg bending its knee and straightening right knee. From this point Form 54 is like Form 12. Body is on a slant forward west. At the same time, continue to move arms: bring right arm forward and place fingertips near left pulse; bend left hand so that fingers point west-downward, with palm north. (Fig. 48)

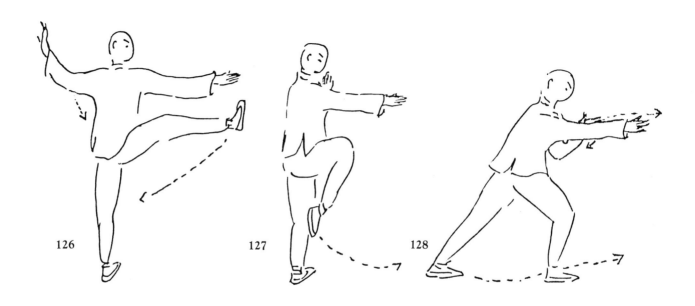

126          127          128

Shift weight back onto right leg, bending right knee, straightening left knee, and flexing foot. At the same time, both arms move: draw right hand back and then down toward right hip bone, gradually making a fist of it. Right elbow points to north; right shoulder contracts, fist-palm is turned upward. While right arms moves, angle left hand so that fingers point upward-west. (Fig. 49, l)

Shift weight forward onto left leg, bending its knee and straightening right knee. At the same time, both arms move: move right arm up west in line with right shoulder, with fist-palm facing south: elbow is straight. Move left palm near inner side of right elbow: wrist is bent with fingers pointing upward. Arm movements and shifting of weight go together. (Fig. 49, 2)

### Form 55. As If You Were Shutting a Door     *Ju Feng Szu Pi*

Same as Form 13. Figures 50, 51
Do not move legs or torso. Move left hand under right arm to its outer side, and turn palm to face right elbow. (Fig. 50)

Shift weight back onto right leg, bending right knee, and straighten left knee, flexing foot. At the same time, both arms move: bend right elbow, bringing fist in toward left shoulder, opening fist gradually so that right palm faces left shoulder, and move left palm facing inward, in to face right shoulder. Left arm is on the outside of right arm. Both elbows are bent downward and forearms are crossed on a diagonal.

At the same time both arms move: move right hand in front of right shoulder with palm facing it and move left hand in front of left shoulder with palm facing it. Elbows are bent downward, wrists are straight, and fingers point upward.

Next, turn both palms to face west, keeping wrists straight and elbows down. All these arm movements are made as weight is shifted from left back onto right leg with bent knee. (Fig. 51)

### Form 56. Carry Tiger To Mountain     *Pao Hu Kuei Shan*

Same as Form 14, Figures 52, 53
Shift weight forward onto left leg, bending knee and straightening right knee. At the same time, push both hands, which are facing west, forward shoulder high to west, each arm in line with its shoulder: wrists are shoulder high; body slants forward on a diagonal west. (Fig. 52)

Keep weight on left leg. Bend torso down, contracting pelvis, moving arms at same time; lower arms so that palms face floor at knee level. Arms are perpendicular to floor. (Fig. 53)

**Form 57. Cross Hands**    *Shih Tsu Shou*

Same as Form 15, Figures 54, 55, 56

Turn right toes to north, and at the same time shift weight onto right leg, bending its knee and straightening left knee. With these movements, torso moves to north, still remaining bent over. At the same time as torso and right toes move, move right hand to right side of right leg, keeping palm facing down; right fingers now point east. Left hand remains at left side; palm is down with fingers pointing west. (Fig. 54)

Gradually raise torso to an upright position, bringing arms up sideways shoulder high, straightening wrists; therefore, palms face downward. Then move arms forward north, shoulder high; at same time turn left toes north. (Fig. 55)

Keeping right knee bent, place left foot parallel to right and apart from it, in your basic stance. Both knees are bent. At the same time as leg moves, bring both arms inward, crossing forearms diagonally: right forearm is on the outside of left; left palm faces east on a slant, right palm faces west on a slant. The cross of the arms is a little below chin level about eight inches away from the face. Elbows are high; back is straight. (Fig. 56)

**Form 58. Oblique Brush Knee Twist Step**    *Hsieh Lou Hsi Niu Pu*

Same as Form 16, to northwest on right side

Move heel of right foot outward to southeast, keeping weight on right leg with its bent knee. This movement releases weight from left leg, and turns torso to face northwest. (Fig. 129)

Move left leg to northwest, straightening knee and flexing foot. Place left heel in the Empty Step Space. Then transfer weight onto left leg, bending knee and straightening right knee. Body slants foward northwest. At the same time both arms move: move right arm forward northwest in line with right shoulder, turning palm to face northwest, and move left arm with bent wrist downward in front of left thigh; fingers point northwest and palm is down. (Fig. 57)

Toe-Heel-Heel-Step

Same as Figures 58-1, 2, 3, 4

Keeping weight on left leg with its bent knee, move left toes inward to point northeast. Straighten torso. At the same time both arms begin to move: move left hand upward with fingers leading with elbows low and move right hand inward toward body at chest level. (Fig. 58-1)

Keeping weight on left leg with its bent knee, move right heel inward, making right foot parallel to left, and bend right knee, so that toes of both feet point northeast. Weight is still on left leg, and torso is straight. At the same time, continue to move both hands toward center of body, with left hand approaching right wrist. (Fig. 58-2)

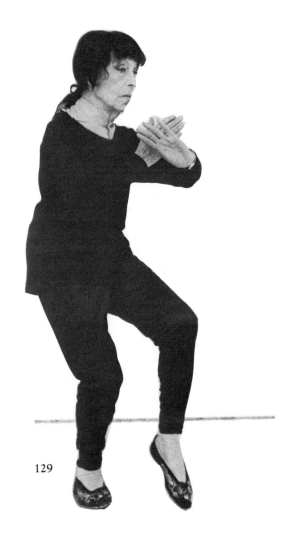

129

Keeping weight on left leg with its bent knee, move left heel outward to northwest. With this movement torso faces east and right knee straightens. Feet are now in T position. At the same time, arms move: continue to move left hand to right wrist, with left fingers pointing southeast; right wrist is bent. (Fig. 58-3)

Weight is still on left leg with its bent knee. Turning torso to face southeast, raise right toes off floor. At the same time, both arms move: move right arm with bent wrist toward front of chest and move left hand over right wrist. (Fig. 58-4)

Oblique Brush Knee Twist Step
To southeast on left side

Place right heel to southeast in the Empty Step Space. Transfer weight onto right leg, bending knee and straightening left knee. Body slants southeast on a diagonal. At the same time, both arms move: move left arm to southeast in line with left shoulder, turning palm to face southeast, and move right hand down to front of right thigh, with palm facing floor and fingers pointing southeast. (Opposite of Figure 57)

**Form 59. Grasping the Bird's Tail**     *Lan Ch'üen Wei*

Same as Form 17, (First) Figures 25, 26, 27, 28, 29, as qualified.

Shift weight back onto left leg, bending knee, straightening right knee, and flexing foot. At the same time both arms move: bring right arm up to southeast, chest high, with palm facing northeast, and place left fingers at right pulse. (Fig. 25, except that here you face southeast instead of east).

Keep the relationship of hands the same. Bending both elbows downward and slightly out, draw both arms inward toward body at chest level, nine inches away from it.

Turn right palm up and left palm down. As hands move, angle left hand so that it is at right angles to right wrist; therefore, left elbow points to northeast. (Fig. 26, except that here you face southeast)

Grasping the Bird's Tail (Second)

Transfer weight onto right leg, bending knee and straightening left knee, with body on a slant to southeast. At the same time as you transfer weight, stretch right arm to east shoulder high, straightening elbow. Keep left fingers above right pulse. (Fig. 27, except that here you face southeast.)

Move both arms in a horizontal circle shoulder high, from east, to southeast, to south, and to west. When arms reach south, bend right elbow downward and bend wrist so that palm faces upward. Turn right fingers to point west. Left arm is adjusted to movements of right arm, because left fingers remain near right pulse.

As you move arms from south, shift weight onto left leg, bending its knee, and straighten right, flexing foot. (Figure 28, except here you face southeast).

Pivot on right heel turning toes to northeast. At the same time, raise right arm with palm up, arcing it upward head high over and down to northeast, straightening arm as you do so, and stop at place where right wrist is slightly above shoulder height. (Fig. 29)

As you are approaching this last position place toes on floor, bend right knee, placing weight on right leg. Bend right wrist, and lower right hand downward so that fingers point downward. As hand bends down place all fingers close together over the thumb as if grasping it. Right arm remains in its position when wrist bends and fingers move. Left fingers are still at right pulse, with palm toward the face. Left wrist is straight and arm is curved. (Fig. 130)

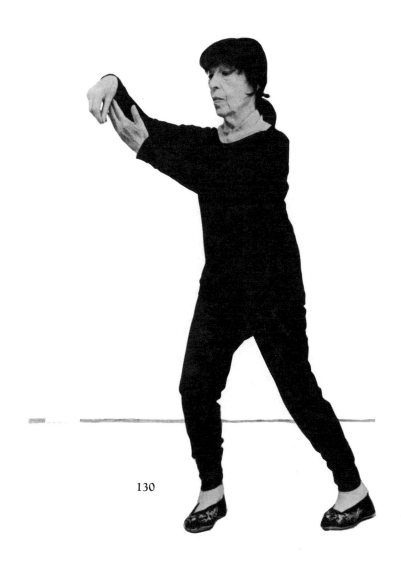

130

### Form 60. The Single Whip (To North)    *Tan Pien*

Same as Form 5, except that here you finish facing *north*, Figures 30, 31
Holding weight on right leg, draw left foot with loose ankle close to right
foot, not touching floor. Then move left foot to west, straightening knee,
and place left foot parallel to right foot. Body is on slant to northeast.
While moving leg, move left arm in a downward curve, in toward body
chest high; then move it up to northwest. Look at left palm as arm moves
up to northwest. Do not tilt head downward. Head moves from right to
left sides. (Fig. 30)

Pivoting on left heel, turn left toes toward the northwest, at the same
time bending left knee to equal that of right knee. Weight is equal on
both legs. Back is straight and torso faces *north*. While you move left toes,
turn left hand to face northwest. (Fig. 131) You are now looking at back of
left hand. Legs, arm, eyes, and head, finish together. Your torso faces north.
(Fig. 132)

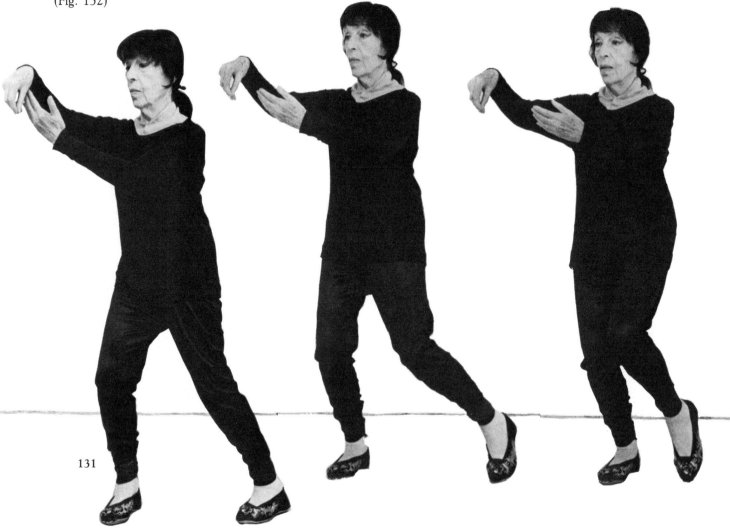

131

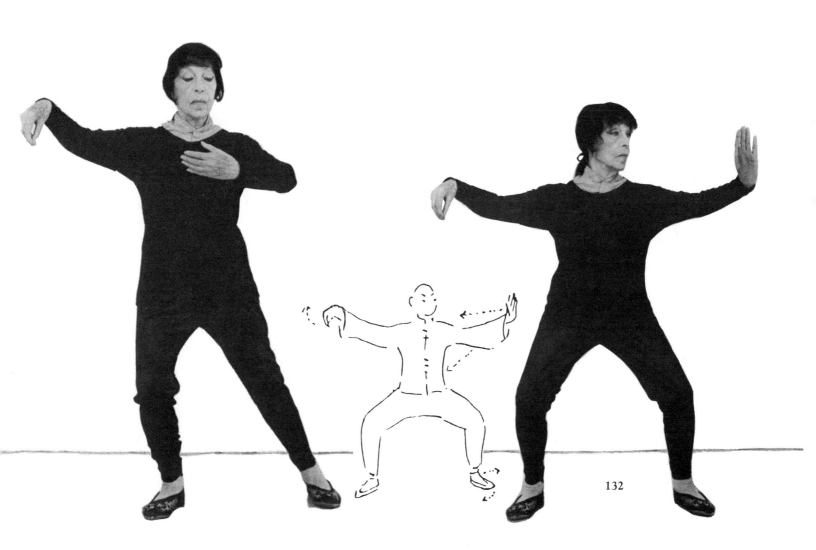

132

**Form 61. Hand Strums the Lute**    *Shou Hui P'i-P'a*

Keep weight on left leg with its bent knee. Move toes of left foot slightly inward and then move left heel outward to west, straightening right knee. At the same time, torso is being turned to face northeast. As you move left toes, both arms move: bending left elbow down, bring hand in toward left shoulder and begin to lift right hand upward. Torso faces northeast. (Fig. 133)

Keeping weight on left leg with its bent knee, raise right toes up, flexing right foot. At the same time, torso is turned to east (Empty Step). With leg and torso movement right hand moves to center in "Lute" position. Simultaneously move left hand forward east and place left fingers at right pulse, palm facing inward. Right palm faces east, with fingers pointing upward. Right foot is flexed, right knee is straight, and right heel touches floor lightly. (Fig. 134)

**Form 62. Parting the Wild Horse's Mane**    *Yeh Ma Fen Tsung*

On right side

Do not move legs. Bend more deeply on left knee and at the same time lean torso from hips diagonally forward and down, keeping back straight. At the same time, both arms move: place left palm above right shoulder, with elbow pointing downward. Straightening right arm, bring it diagonally downward across body, so that left elbow and right inner elbow meet. This movement pulls shoulders forward but *not* up. Right palm faces northwest, with fingers pointing diagonally downward to northeast. Wrists are straight. (Fig. 135)

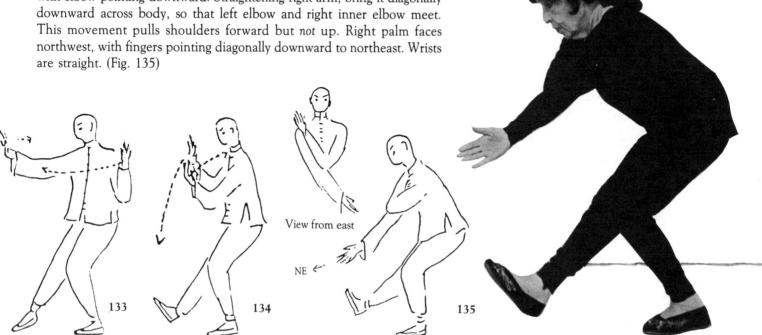

View from east

NE

133    134    135

Keep weight on left leg with its bent knee, and do not move right flexed foot. Lift torso up and turn it to face northeast; hips are even and torso does not slant. At the same time, both arms move: bend right arm upward. Elbows separate as left palm turns outward and right palm inward. Face right palm in front of left shoulder and turn left palm outward to face out opposite right shoulder. Arms are crossed at middle of forearms; right arm is on outside; elbows are squared away from shoulders. (Fig. 136)

Place weight on right leg, bending right knee and straightening left knee. At the same time body and both arms move: body is slanted toward east, keeping head and torso facing northeast. Move right arm forward north at shoulder level, with palm up; continue to move it in a horizontal circle toward east where it stops in line with right shoulder, palm up. Turn left palm to east and, bending wrist, move arm downward and stop hand chest high in space between body and right arm. Head faces northeast. Legs, arms, and body move together. (Fig. 137)

Then, as as separate movement, turn head to east and look at right palm.

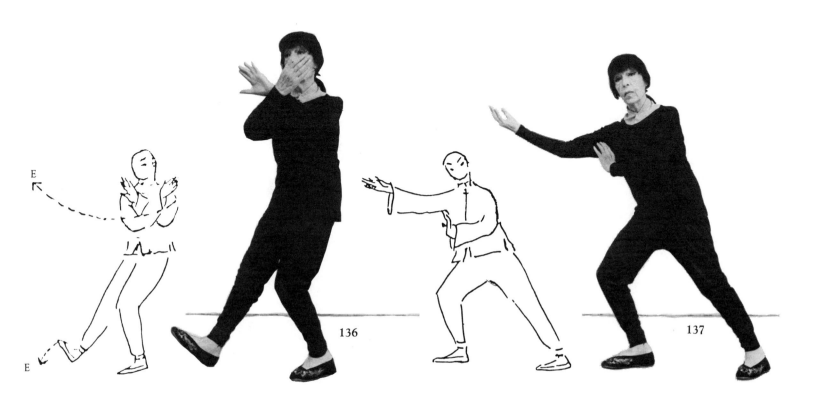

136

137

**Form 63. Hand Strums the Lute**    *Shou Hui P'i-P'a*

Same as Form 61, Figure 134

Turning torso to face east, shift weight back onto left leg, bending its knee, straightening right knee, and flexing right foot. At the same time, both arms move: turn right palm to face east bending elbow downward, and place left fingers at right pulse, palm facing inward. (Fig. 134)

**Form 64. Parting the Wild Horse's Mane**    *Yeh Ma Fen Tsung*

On right side—same as Form 62, Figures 135, 136, 137

Do not move legs. Bend more deeply on left knee and at the same time lean torso from hips, diagonally forward and down; keep back straight. At the same time both arms move: place left palm above right shoulder, with elbow pointing downward opposite chest. Straightening right arm, bring it diagonally downward across body, so that left elbow and right inner elbow meet. This movement pulls shoulders forward. Right palm faces northwest with fingers pointing diagonally downward to northeast; wrists are straight. (Fig. 135)

Keep weight on left with its bent knee and do not move right flexed foot. Lift torso up and turn it to face northeast; hips are even and torso does not slant. At the same time, both arms move: bend right arm upward; elbows separate as left palm turns outward. Face right palm in front of left shoulder, and turn left palm to face northeast keeping left hand opposite right shoulder. Arms are crossed at middle of forearms; elbows are squared away from shoulders. (Fig. 136)

Place weight on right leg, bending right knee and straightening left knee. At the same time body and both arms move: slant body toward east and keep head and torso northeast. Move right arm forward north with palm up; continue to move it in a horizontal circle toward the east where the arm stops level in line with right shoulder. Palm is up. Turn left palm to east, and bending wrist, move arm downward and stop hand chest high in the space between body and right arm. Head faces northeast. (Fig. 135)

Then, as separate movement, turn head to east and look at right palm. (Fig. 138-139)

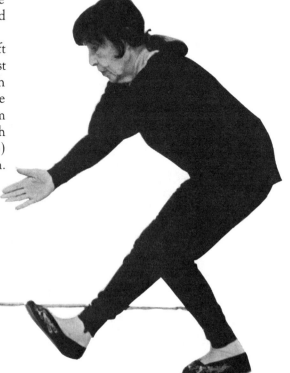

135

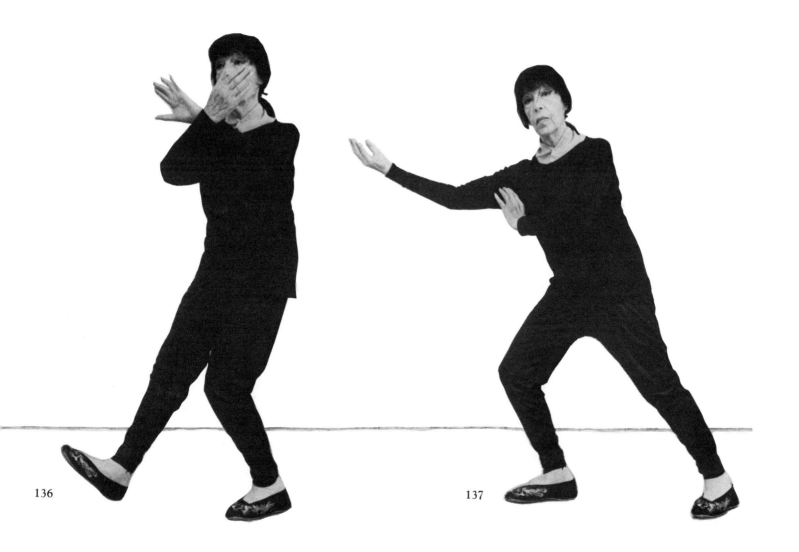

136                                                    137

Parting the Wild Horse's Mane

On left side

Turn head so that you are looking southeast, do *not* move rest of body. (Fig. 139)

Keep weight on right leg, with slant of body diagonally to east. Turn torso to face east, as Figure 139 shows. At the same time as torso moves, place right palm above left shoulder, bending elbow downward. Straightening left arm, bring it diagonally downward across body so that right elbow and left inner elbow meet away from chest—at chest level. Left palm faces southwest, with fingers pointing diagonally to southeast. Wrists are straight. The direction of torso is east; head is southeast, weight is forward on right leg. (Fig. 140)

Draw left foot close to right foot, not touching floor. Place left heel forward east in Empty Step. At the same time, cross arms and turn torso to southeast. Bend left arm upward, keeping elbow even with right elbow. Face left palm opposite right shoulder, and turn right palm outward to face southeast, keeping hand in front of left shoulder. Arms are crossed at middle of forearms, left arm is on the outside, and elbows are apart. (Fig. 141)

Transfer weight onto left leg, bending its knee and straightening right knee. Head remains looking southeast, torso faces southeast, and body slants forward east. At the same time, both arms move: move left arm to south at shoulder level, with palm up, and continue to move it in a horizontal circle toward east where arm stops at shoulder level in line with left shoulder. Palm is up. Turn right palm east and bending wrist, move hand downward and stop hand chest high in space between body and left arm. Legs, arms, and body move and finish at the same time. Head is facing southeast. (Fig. 142)

Then, as a separate movement, turn head to east and look at left palm.

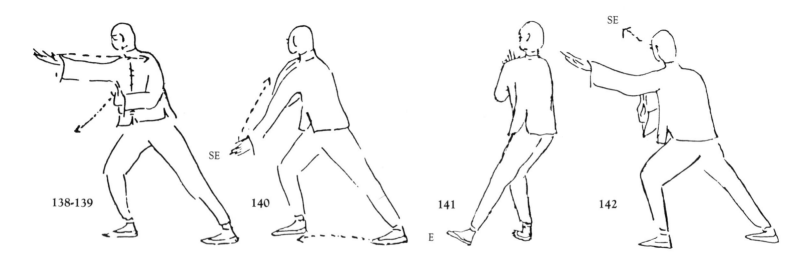

138-139　　　　　　140　　　　　　141　　　　　　142

On right side—same as Form 62, Figures 136, 137

Turn head so that you are looking northeast; do not move body. (Fig. 143) Keep weight on left leg, with diagonal slant of body to east. Turn torso to face east, head remains looking northeast. At the same time as torso moves, place left palm opposite right shoulder, bending elbow. Straightening right arm, bring it diagonally downward across body so that left elbow and right inner elbow meet opposite chest. Right palm faces northwest with fingers pointing diagonally downward to northeast. Wrists are straight.

Draw right foot close to left foot, not touching floor; place right foot forward east in the Empty Step Space. At the same time, cross arms and turn torso to face northeast. Bend right arm upward, keeping elbow even with left elbow. Face right palm opposite left shoulder, and turn left palm to face north keeping hand opposite right shoulder. Arms are crossed at middle of forearms; right arm is on the outside; elbows are apart. Right leg, arms and torso move and finish positions at the same time. (Reverse of Figure 141)

Transfer weight onto right leg, bending its knee and straightening left knee. Head remains looking northeast, torso faces northeast, and body slants to east. At the same time move both arms: move right arm forward to north with palm up; continue to move it in a horizontal circle toward

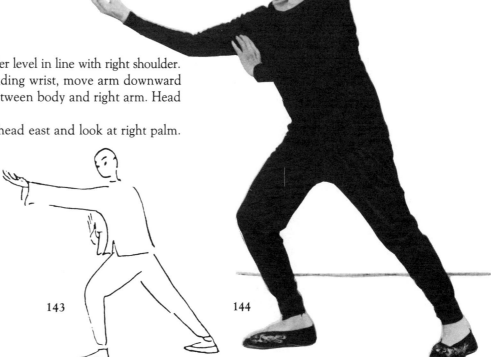

the east where the arm stops above shoulder level in line with right shoulder. Palm is up. Turn left palm east, and bending wrist, move arm downward and stop hand chest high in the space between body and right arm. Head faces northeast. (Fig. 144)

Then, as a separate movement, turn head east and look at right palm.

143     144

**Form 65. Hand Strums the Lute**     *Shou Hui P'i-P'a*

Same as Form 63, Figure 134

Turn torso to face east and shift weight back onto left leg bending its knee, straightening right knee and flexing right foot (Empty Step). At the same time, both arms move: turn right palm to face east, bending elbow downward, and place left fingers at right pulse, palm facing inward nine inches from chest. (Fig. 134)

**Form 66. Parting the Wild Horse's Mane**     *Yeh Ma Fen Tsung*

Same as Form 62, Figures 135, 136, 137. Do not omit.

Do not move feet. Bend more deeply on left knee and at the same time lean torso from hips diagonally forward and down. Keep back straight. At the same time both arms move: place left palm above right shoulder with elbow pointing downward. Straighten right arm and bring it diagonally downward across body, so that left elbow and right inner elbow meet at chest level. Right palm faces northwest, with fingers pointing toward floor to northeast. Wrists are straight. (Fig. 135)

   Keep weight on left with its bent knee and do not move right flexed foot. Lift torso up and turn it to face northeast; hips are even and torso does not slant. At the same time both arms move: bend right arm upward, keeping elbow even with left elbow. Face right palm opposite left shoulder and turn left palm to face north, keeping hand opposite right shoulder. (Fig. 136)

   Place weight on right leg, bending its knee and straightening left knee. Move arms and body at the same time: slant torso east and keep torso and head facing northeast. Move right arm forward north with palm up; continue to move it in a horizontal circle toward the east where the arm stops above shoulder level in line with right shoulder. Palm is up. Turn left palm to east and bending wrist, move arm downward, stopping hand chest high between body and right arm. Head faces north. (Fig. 137)

   Then, as a separate movement, turn head to east and look at right palm.

**Form 67. Jade Girl (Angel) Works at the Shuttle**     *Yü Nü Ch'üan So*

On left side facing east

Keep weight on right leg. Draw left foot with loose ankle close to right foot not touching floor, and turn torso to east. At the same time both arms move: place right palm above left shoulder with elbow shoulder high, and lower left arm, placing it in front of body, abdomen high, with palm down and fingers pointing south. Left arm is curved with elbow pointing north. (Fig. 145)

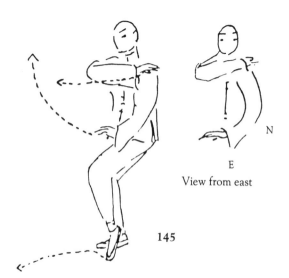

N

E

View from east

145

Place left heel forward east in the Empty Step space; transfer weight onto left leg, bending its knee and straightening right knee. Body slants east. At the same time move arms: raise left curved arm up east (elbow points north) so that arm is at shoulder level: palm faces east. Bend wrist sideways up, making hand slant upward slightly, 15 inches from face. Move right hand near left forearm with palm facing east, and place right fingertips two inches from left wrist: right wrist is bent and elbow points down. In this relationship, right finger-tips are at mouth level, 15 inches from mouth. (Fig. 146)

Keep body on a slant. Do not move legs. Keeping arms and head in same relationship to body, twist at waist and move upper torso to face north. (Fig. 147)

Then move torso to east.

Now move torso to southeast. (Fig. 148)

Again move torso back to east. During this waist-circling movement do not change position of head. (Fig. 146)

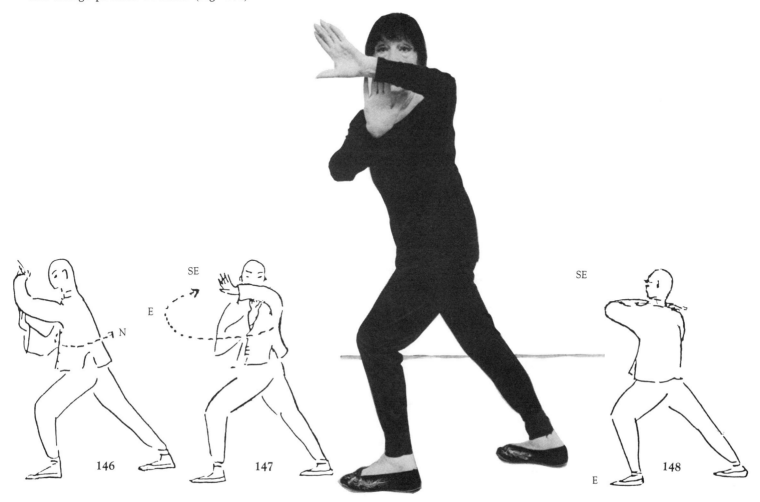

146    147    148

**Form 68. Jade Girl (Angel) Works at the Shuttle**    *Yü Nü Ch'üan So*

On right side facing west

Keeping weight on left leg, turn toes of left foot to south; turn right heel inward making foot parallel to left with weight on left; next turn left heel out to east and straighten right knee: then flex right foot. While you do this Toe-Heel-Heel-step and are turning torso to face west, both arms move: place left palm above right shoulder with elbow shoulder high, and lower right arm curved downward with palm facing floor, placing it in front of body, abdomen high. (Fig. 149)

Place right heel forward west in Empty Step Space; transfer weight onto right leg, bending its knee and straightening left knee. Body slants forward west. At the same time both arms move: raise right arm curved up west so that arm is at shoulder level; palm faces west and wrist bends sideways-up, making hand slant upward slightly, 15 inches from face. Move left hand near right forearm with palm facing west, and place fingertips two inches from right wrist; left wrist is bent and elbow points down; fingertips are opposite mouth. (Fig. 150)

Do not move legs. Keep body on a slant. Keeping arms and head in same relationship to body, twist at waist and move upper torso to face north.

Then move torso to face west.

Then move torso to face southwest.

Now move torso back to west. During this waist circling movement do not change position of head. (Fig. 150)

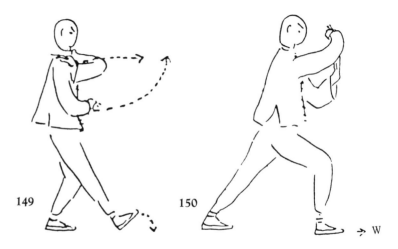

149          150          → W

**Form 69. Hand Strums the Lute**     *Shou Hui P'i-P'a*

Same as Form 63, except that here you face *west*.

Shift weight back onto left leg, bending its knee and straightening right knee, and flexing foot. At the same time, both arms move: move right arm a bit inward bending elbow downward; keep palm facing west, with fingers pointing upward. Place left fingers at right pulse, facing left palm inward nine inches from chest. (Fig. 151)

**Form 70. Parting the Wild Horse's Mane**     *Yeh Ma Fen Tsng*

On right side—same as Form 62, Figures 135, 136, 137, except that here you face west.

Do not move legs. Bend more deeply on left knee and at the same time, lean torso from hips, forward and diagonally down. Keep back straight. At the same time arms move: place left palm above right shoulder, with elbow pointing downward. Straightening right arm, bring it diagonally downward across body so that left elbow and right inner elbow meet opposite chest. Right palm faces southeast with fingers pointing toward floor to southwest. Wrists are straight. (Fig. 135)

Keep weight on left leg with its bent knee, and do not move right flexed foot. Lift torso up and turn it to face southwest; hips are even and torso does not slant. At the same time, both arms move: bend right arm upward, keeping elbow even with left elbow. Face right palm opposite left shoulder and turn left palm outward to face southwest; elbows are down and apart. (Fig. 136)

Place weight on right leg, bending right knee and straightening left knee. Slant body toward west, and keep torso and head facing southwest. Move right arm to south and continue to move it in a horizontal circle toward west where arm stops in line with right shoulder. Palm is up. Turn left palm west, and bending wrist, move arm downward and stop hand chest high in space between body and right arm. Head faces southwest. Legs, body, and both arms all move together. (Fig. 137)

Then, as a separate movement, turn head to west and look at right palm.

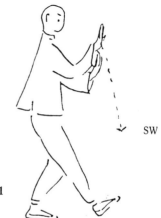

SW

151

**Form 71. Jade Girl (Angel) Works at the Shuttle**   *Yü Nü Ch'üan So*

Left side, facing west, Figures 145, 146, 147, 148

Keep weight on right leg. Draw left foot with loose ankle to right foot not touching floor, and turn torso west. At the same time both arms move: place right palm above left shoulder with elbow shoulder high and lower left arm, placing it in front of body abdomen-high-palm facing floor, with fingers pointing north. Left elbow points south. (Fig. 145)

Place left heel forward west, in the Empty Step Space; transfer weight onto left leg, bending knee and straightening right knee. Body is on a slant west. At the same time, both arms move: raise left curved arm up west (elbow is south) so that arm is at shoulder level: palm faces west, and wrist bends sideways-up, making hand slant upward slightly. Move right hand near left forearm and place fingertips two inches from left wrist; right palm faces west; wrist is bent, and elbow points down. (Fig. 146, except that here you face west as in Figure 152.) Fingertips are at mouth level.

Keep body on a slant. Do not move legs, keeping arms and head in same relationship to body; twist at waist and move upper torso to face south.

Then move torso to face west.

Then move torso to northwest.

Now move torso to west. During this waist-circling movement do not change position of head. (Fig. 152)

**Form 72. Jade Girl (Angel) Works at the Shuttle**   *Yü Nü Ch'üan So*

On right side, but this time you face east

Keep weight on left leg. Turn toes of left to point north; move right heel inward making foot parallel to left foot; turn left heel outward to west and straighten right knee; then flex right foot. While you do this Toe-Heel-Heel step, and are turning torso to east, both arms move: place left palm above right shoulder with elbow shoulder high and lower right curved arm downward with palm facing floor, body abdomen-high. (Fig. 153)

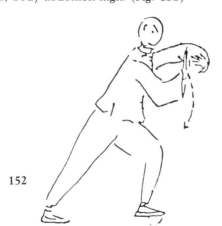

152

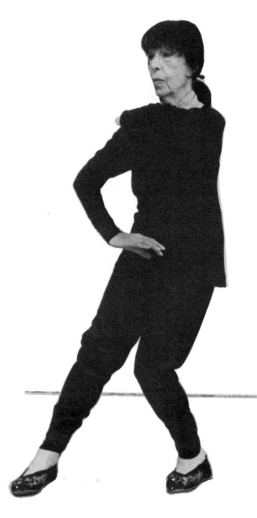

153

Place right heel forward to east in the Empty Step Space; transfer weight onto right leg, bending its knee and straightening left knee. Body is on a slant to east. Both arms move at the same time as leg moves: raise curved right arm up to east at shoulder level, point elbow south, and face palm to east. Wrist bends sideways-up so that hand is slanted upward slightly. Move left hand near right forearm and place finger tips two inches from right wrist. Palm faces east. Left wrist is bent and elbow points down. Finger tips are at mouth level.

Do not move legs. Keep body on a slant. Keeping arms and head in same relationship to body, twist at waist and move upper torso to face south.

Then move torso to face east.

Then move torso to face northeast. (Fig. 153 and 154)

Then move torso to face east. (Fig. 155) During this waist-circling movement, do not change position of head.

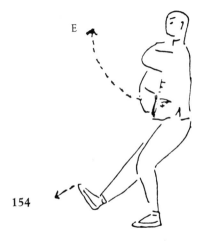

**154**

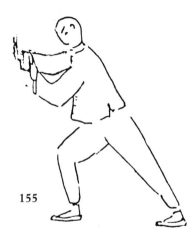

**155**

**Form 73. Hand Strums the Lute**     *Shou Hui P'i-P'a*

Facing east, same as Form 63, Figure 134

Shift weight back onto left leg, bending knee, straightening right knee and flexing foot. At the same time, both arms move: move right arm bending elbow downward, keeping palm east with right fingers pointing upward. Place left fingers at right pulse with left palm facing inward 9 inches from chest. (Fig 134)

**Form 74. Parting the Wild Horse's Mane**     *Yeh Ma Fen Tsung*

On right side, Form 62, Figures 135, 136, 137

Do not move feet. Bend more deeply on left knee and at the same time lean torso diagonally forward and down. At the same time both arms move: place left palm above right shoulder with elbow pointing downward. Straightening right arm, bring it diagonally across body so that left elbow and right inner elbow meet. Right palm faces northwest with fingers pointing toward floor to northeast. Wrists are straight. (Fig. 135)

Keep weight on left leg with its bent knee, and do not move right flexed foot. Lift torso up and turn it to face northeast. At the same time, both arms move: bend right arm upward and place palm above left shoulder, and turn left palm outward to face northeast, keeping hand opposite right shoulder. Arms are crossed at middle of forearms, the right on the outside, with elbows squared and apart.

Place weight on right foot, bending right knee and straightening left knee. At the same time body and both arms move: slant body to east, keeping torso and head facing northeast. Move right arm north at shoulder level with palm up; continue to move it in a horizontal circle toward east where arm stops in line with right shoulder. Turn left palm to east, and bending wrist, move arm downward and stop hand chest high in space between upper right arm and body. Head faces northeast. Leg, body, and arms move together. (Fig. 137)

Then, as a separate movement, turn head to east and look at right palm.

# Form 75. Grasping the Bird's Tail   *Lan Ch'üeh Wei*

Same as Forms 2, 3, 4, Figures 25, 26, 27, 28, 29

Shift weight back onto left leg, bending its knee, straightening right knee, and flexing foot (Empty Step). At the same time, move both arms: placing left finger tips at right pulse, keep right fingers pointing east, turning right palm to face north, and turn left palm to face south: both elbows are curved downward. Hands are at chest level. (Fig. 25)

Keeping the relationship of hands the same, move both arms inward toward body at chest level, bending both elbows downward and slightly out; right wrist within nine inches of chest.

Turn right palm up bending wrist and left palm down at the same time. As you move hands, angle left hand so that it is at right angles to right wrist, so that left elbow points north. (Fig. 26)

Shift weight onto right leg, bending its knee and straightening left knee. Body is on slant forward east. At the same time, stretch right arm to northeast, straightening right elbow. Left fingers remain at right pulse. Arms are shoulder level high. (Fig. 27)

Circle both arms horizontally, shoulder high, from northeast, to east, to southeast. When arms reach southeast bend right elbow downward and bend right wrist so that palm faces upward. With fingers leading the movement, right fingers point southwest at the end of this horizontal circling. Left arm is adjusted to movement of the right, because left fingers always remain near right pulse. (Fig. 28)

As you bend right elbow from southeast, shift weight back onto left leg, bending its knee, straightening right knee, and flexing right foot. (Fig. 28)

Pivot on right heel, to northeast, flexing foot. At same time, raise right arm with palm leading up arcing head high over and down toward northeast, straightening right arm as you do so, and stop in position where right wrist is slightly above shoulder height. (Fig. 29)

As you are approaching this last arm position and place toes on floor, bend right knee, placing weight on right leg and straightening left knee. Then bend right wrist and lower hand making fingers point downward in Grasping position. Right arm remains in place while hand moves. Left fingers remain near right pulse, with palm facing you. (Fig. 29)

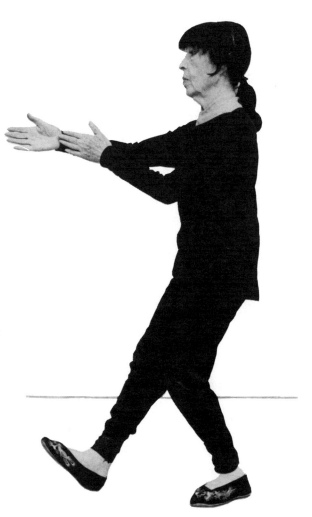

### Form 76. The Single Whip    *Tan Pien*

Same as Form 5, Figures 30 and 31

Hold weight on right leg with its bent knee. Draw left foot with loose ankle close to right one, not touching floor. Then move left leg backward to southwest diagonal in the Walking Step Space, Straighten left knee and place foot parallel to right foot. Weight is on right leg; body is on a slant to northeast. As left leg moves, move left arm with palm toward face in a downward curve, circling in toward body waist high. Left arm is curved and palm is toward your face, chest high eight inches away from it. Right arm does not move. (Fig. 30)

Pivoting on left heel, turn toes toward the northwest. Place weight on left leg and bend left knee to equal that of right knee. Now your weight is even on both legs. Body is turned to northwest. Feet are separated by a distance equal to twice the length of your foot. Your back is straight.

As left foot moves, turn left palm to face the northwest. Now both arms are on the same level, with wrists higher than shoulder level. (Fig. 31)

Keep looking at left palm as hand moves to northwest. Move head from right to left sides. Do not bend head when eyes look downward. When left palm turns to northwest, you will then be looking at the back of left hand.

Synchronize movements of eyes, arm, legs, head, and body. (Figure 156)

### Form 77. Cloud Arms    *Yün Shou*

Same as Form 32, Figures 87, 88, 89, 90, 91. Do not omit (see page 74). Do not move right arm. Turn left toes inward to point north and then move left heel outward to make foot parallel to right foot. With the movements of left foot, shift weight onto right leg and straighten left knee: body slants to northeast. At the same time as you move left foot and shift weight, circle left arm downward and then inward to body, abdomen high, keeping wrist bent. Gradually straightening wrist, move left arm upwards toward right wrist. Place left fingers near right pulse, with palm inward facing you. As left arm moves, raise right hand slowly upward, opening hand to face palm northeast. Left foot, left arm, and right hand move together. (Fig. 87)

Shift weight back onto left leg, bending left knee and straightening right knee. At the same time, both arms move: looking at left palm, move left arm with palm at eye level, twelve inches away from face. Keep eyes fixed on palm. At the same time, circle right arm outward to right side, and then downward, with bent wrist and palm facing down. (Fig. 88)

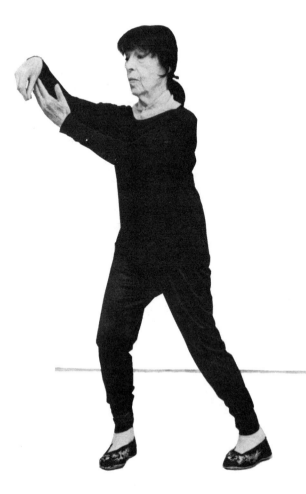

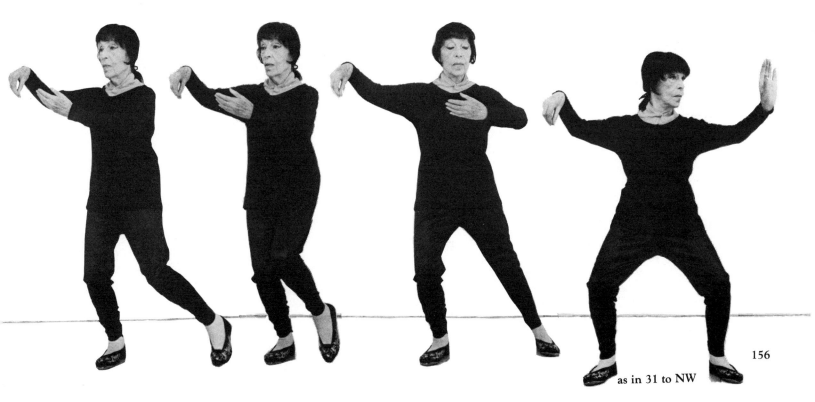

156

as in 31 to NW

Turn torso north, keeping weight on left leg. Turn right toes inward to point northwest. Then turn left toes outward to point northwest. As toes move, torso moves to face northwest. Along with feet and torso, both arms move: continue to move left arm, face high, to left side, with eyes looking at palm. Continue to move right arm in its circle from downward to inward abdomen high in front of body, gradually straightening wrist. Then move hand upward toward left hand. (Fig. 89)

Keeping weight on left leg, place right foot parallel and apart from left in your basic stance: both toes point northwest; both knees are evenly bent; back is straight; torso faces northwest. Both arms continue to move: turn left palm to face northwest, at eye level, while you move right fingers up to left pulse, turning right palm to face your face. Look at right palm now. Both elbows point downward. (Fig. 90)

Turn torso toward right to face north and move right arm to right side, with palm at eye level, twelve inches away from face. Eyes look at right palm. Then turn right toes to point northeast, placing weight onto right leg with its bent knee. Then turn left knee inward, touching left toes to floor with loose ankle, thus taking most weight off left foot. At the same time as right arm and torso turn to north, move left arm: move left arm with wrist bent and palm out, outward to left shoulder side, and then downward. Continue to circle it inward to body abdomen high, gradually straightening wrist. Then move it up toward the right pulse. (Fig. 91)

As left hand goes upward toward right side, place left leg diagonally backward to southwest in the Walking Step Space. Straighten left knee and keep right knee with weight on right leg. Body slants to northeast. On this last movement, turn right palm out to face northeast, and place left fingers at right pulse with palm toward face. Eyes look far away to northeast while left hand, right hand, left foot, and shifting eye gaze are made simultaneously. (Fig. 87)

*Repeat* all of Cloud Arms from Figure 87. Go to 88, 89, 90, 91, and 87 again in exactly the same way. Do not omit this repeat (See page 75)


## Form 78. The Single Whip     *Tan Pien*

Same as Form 5, Figures 30 and 31

Continue this from the repeat of Figure 87. Bend right wrist downward and place fingers down in grasping position. Then move left arm downward, and inward toward chest. (Fig. 30)

Continue left arm upward, northwest. Turn left palm to face northwest and turn left toes also to northwest; bend left knee to equal that of right knee. Back is straight. As left arm moves, look at palm as it moves downward and upward. Move head from right to left side. Look at back of left hand on its last movement. Torso faces northwest. (Fig. 31)

**Form 79. The Snake Creeps Down**    *She Shen Hsia Shih*

Turn left palm upward, as weight is shifting gradually to left leg, straightening right knee and lifting right heel off floor. As weight shifts move both arms: bend left elbow shoulder high bringing hand to head level, wrist bent and palm up; hand is vertically above elbow which is in a right angle bend. Right arm moves after left hand has turned palm up: bending elbow shoulder high lift right hand up and bring it a little above forehead, palm up. Fingers of both hands point west and are twelve inches apart. (Fig. 157)

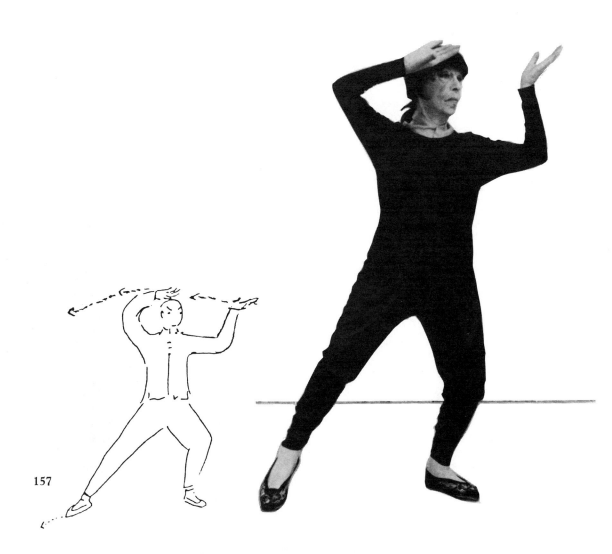

157

Do not move arms. *Quickly* step right leg out to northeast on a diagonal, bending knee slightly and straightening left leg. Then move both hands with palms up around to south, then southeast; then right hand moves to northeast, palm up at head level, straightening elbow; while left hand with palm up moves to forehead. With the ending of the arm movements, turn right toes out to northeast. Torso remains northwest. (Fig. 158)

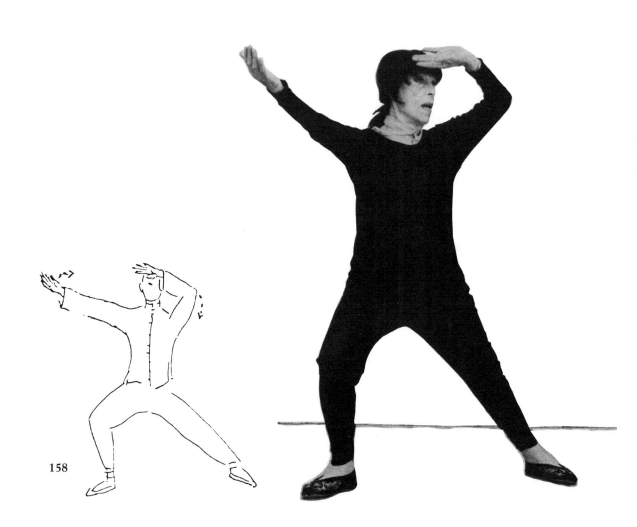

158

Keep weight on right leg. Turn left hand outward, then bend wrist so that fingers point north and palm east, all the while lowering arm to chest level, five inches away. Left elbow is on a horizontal line with left wrist. At same time, bend right wrist so that palm faces inward and fingers point diagonally down. Move hand in a southwest path to shoulder level, slightly in front of it. Right elbow is higher than hand. (Fig. 159)

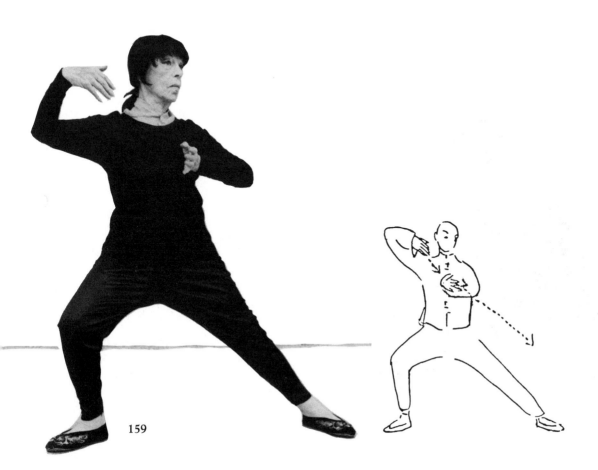

159

Arms, torso and right knee bend all move together: turn torso northwest and then bend it forward northwest. Move left hand, straightening wrist, finger-tips, leading diagonally downward to northwest; right hand, straightening wrist, moves on a southwest path and fingers stop at left elbow joint, palm inward. Both wrists are straight; head and torso are northwest. While all movements go toward northwest, keep lowering the right knee bend. The torso will therefore be weighted toward the right side, even though it is bending forward and facing toward the left, northwest direction. (Fig. 160)

### Form 80. Golden Cockerel Stands on One Leg    *Chin Chi Tu Li*
Right side
Shift weight onto left leg, bending its knee. At the same time, both arms move: start to raise left arm up to left with fingers to west, and move right arm vertically downward with fingers pointing to floor. Wrists are straight. (Fig. 161)

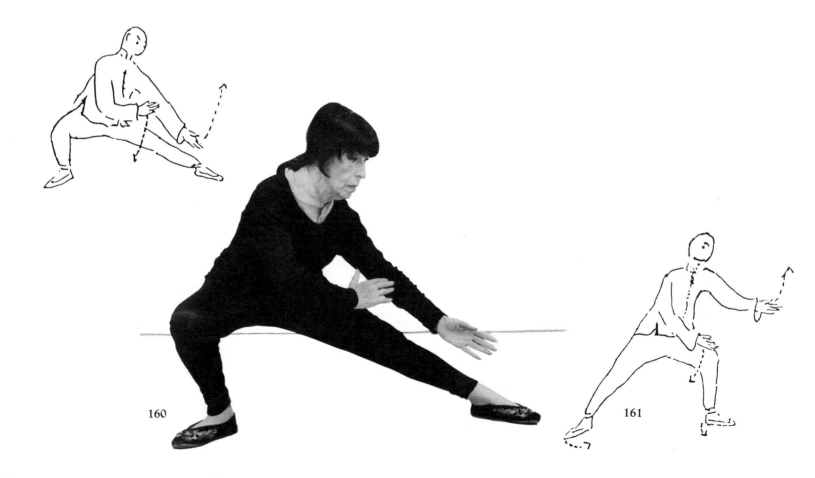

160

161

At the same time as arms move, turn right toes to point northwest, straightening right knee. Then move left heel inward to make foot point west; weight is on left leg with its bent knee. The movements of right toes and left heel turn torso to face west. Body is on a slant forward west. While you shift toes and heel, complete the movements of arms. Move left arm upward in line with left shoulder, with palm north and fingers west; and move right arm downward vertically at right side, with palm inward toward body and fingers pointing downward. (Fig. 162)

Shift all weight onto the left: draw right foot with loose ankle to left foot, not touching floor; torso is vertical, leg is straight. Then raise right leg up high toward west: right knee is high and lower part of leg is held high, with flexed foot. At the same time, both arms move: move right arm toward west, shoulder high and then circle it inward toward forehead. Turn back of hand to forehead: palm faces west, elbow is curved and points north. Move left arm in a curve inward to meet right knee: place hand with palm west above right knee: elbow points south. Right leg and both arms move and finish movements together. Left knee is straight. Torso is slightly curved forward. (Fig. 163)

**Form 81. Golden Cockerel Stands on One Leg**      *Chin Chi Tu Li*
Left side
Bend right knee and bring right foot with loose ankle close to left knee. At the same time, both arms move: circle right arm outward west with palm out, and circle it downward and inward. Place right hand under left hand, which remains at right knee level. At the same time as right palm goes under it, turn left palm to face upward. Right palm faces knee. Backs of hands are toward each other, not touching. (Fig. 164)

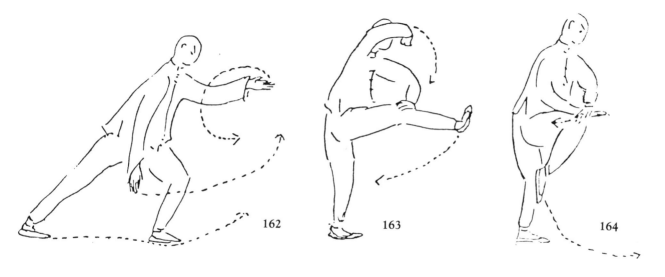

162      163      164

Bending on left leg, place right heel west in the Empty Step Space. Transfer weight onto right leg, bending its knee and straightening left knee. Body slants forward west. Start to move hands when weight is being shifted to right leg. Keeping left hand above right, move both arms out to north, then upward to shoulder height staying to right of torso. (Fig. 165)

Continue to move hands high arced toward forehead. As you do so, draw left foot with loose ankle over to right foot, standing straight on right leg, and start to raise left foot up toward west. (Fig. 166) As you raise left leg, separate hands: circle right arm downward and place right hand above left knee with palm west. At the same time, turn left hand, which is already at forehead, to face palm west. Left leg is now up high to west, knee is bent, and lower leg is high, with foot flexed. (Fig. 167)

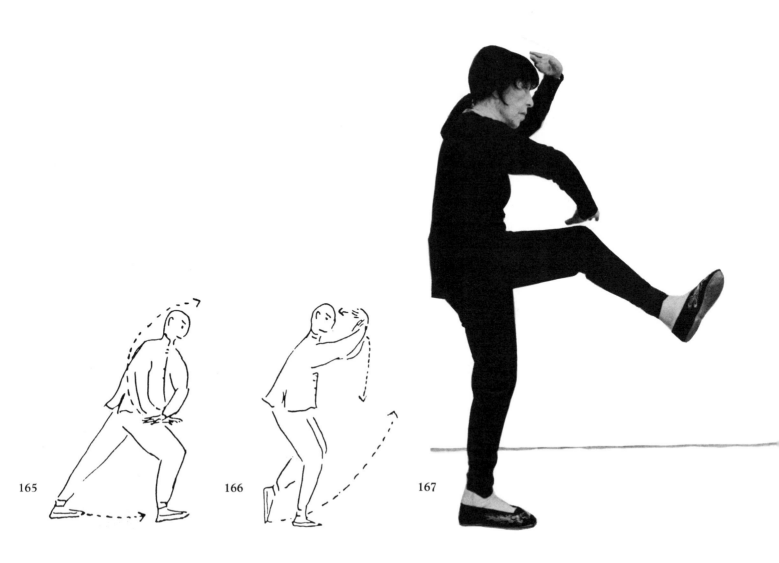

165

166

167

## Form 82. Brush Knee Twist Step    *Lou Hsi Niu Pu*

Backward on left side, similar to Form 20, Figures 66, 67, 68, 44

Bring left elbow down close to body and bend wrist so that fingers point west with palm north: wrist is close to upper left arm. At the same time, bend left knee and move left foot with loose ankle to right knee. Keep right hand above right knee. (Fig. 168)

Bending left knee, lower left foot with loose ankle close to right foot, not touching floor. Gradually move right arm to right. (Fig. 66)

Weight remains on right leg with its bent knee. Place left foot backward to east in the Walking Step Space, and straighten its knee. Body slants forward west. As left leg moves, move left arm forward west in line with left shoulder, turning hand to face west; while right hand finishes its movement at front of right thigh, palm down and fingers pointing west. (Fig. 67)

Brush Knee Twist Step
Going backward on right side

Shift weight back onto left leg, bending its knee; straighten right knee, and flex foot (Empty Step). Move left hand inward to center ten inches from chest, keeping elbow high: palm is west with fingers pointing north. At the same time as leg and left hand move, move right hand upward above left wrist, with fingers pointing west and palm south. (Fig. 68)

Keep weight on left leg with its bent knee. Draw right foot with loose ankle close to left. Then place right foot backward to east in the Walking Step Space, straightening right leg. At the same time, both arms move: move right arm forward west in line with right shoulder, turning palm to west. Circle left arm downward to front of left thigh with palm down and fingers pointing west. (Fig. 169)

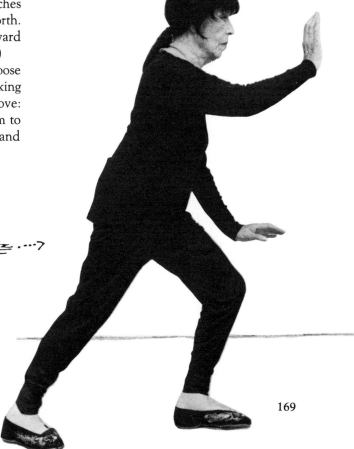

168,1

as in 67

168,2

169

Brush Knee Twist Step
Going backward on left side

Shift weight back onto right leg bending its knee, straighten left knee, and flex foot (Empty Step). Draw right hand inward toward center, ten inches from chest, keeping elbow high: palm faces west and fingers point south. At the same time, move left hand upward above right wrist, with fingers pointing west and palm facing north.

Keep weight on right leg. Without touching floor, draw left foot with loose ankle to right foot. Place left leg backward to east in the Walking Step Space, straightening left knee. Body slants forward west. At the same time, both arms move: move left arm forward west in line with left shoulder, turning palm west, and circle right arm downward to front of right thigh, with palm down and fingers pointing west. (Fig. 67)

**Form 83. Flying Oblique**     *Hsieh Fei Shih*
Same as Form 21, Figures 70, 71, 72, 73
Keep weight on right leg with its bent knee. Foot, hand and head move together. Turn toes right foot to northwest. Turn right palm up, keeping fingers pointing west. Bend head down, and turn chin toward right shoulder. Do not move arms or shoulders; do not shift weight from right leg. Movements are made in ankle, wrist, and neck. (Fig. 70)

(1) Turn torso to northwest; right arm will then be at right side of right leg. (2) Bend torso, bending left knee lower; this releases left leg—knee bends, heel rises with toes on floor. Right hand is at knee level. (Fig. 71) (3) Move left foot inward to right foot. Continue to move left foot outward toward southwest as far as it can go with a straight knee. Place left foot parallel to right foot so that both feet point northwest. At the same time turn right hand with palm up inward to northeast: fingers point to northeast. (Fig. 170)

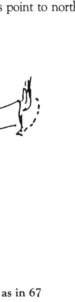

170,1

as in 67

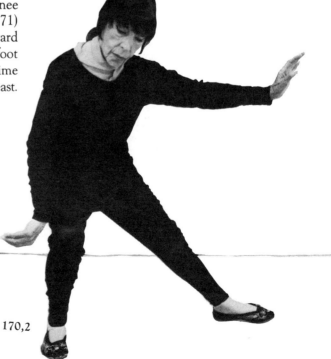

170,2

Shift weight onto left leg, bending its knee, and straighten right knee. Torso is forward and faces northwest; head looks toward northeast. At the same time as weight goes to left leg, turn *left* palm up with fingers pointing west and straighten wrist. At the same time, turn right palm down with fingers pointing to northeast. Right arm is parallel to right leg. Look at back of right hand. All movements finish together. (Fig. 171)

### Form 84. Raise Hands and Step Up   *T'i Shou Shang Shih*

Same as Form 6, Figures 35, 36, 37

Turn right toes to point north and shift weight onto right leg, bending its knee and straightening left knee. On these movements, straighten torso, turn it to face north. Then turn toes of left foot to point north. At same time, turn right palm sideways with straight wrist, lift it up northeast shoulder high. Then curve right elbow bringing right hand over to left side shoulder level, palm inward. As arms move, torso bends forward north.

Move left hand with palm turned to northeast toward inner curve of right elbow. Left elbow points downward and right elbow is chest high. (Fig. 35)

Draw left foot up to right and place it parallel and apart from right foot in your basic stance. Both knees are equally bent and torso is curved forward north. At the same time, arms complete the movements described above: right is curved forward chest high and left palm is at inner curve of right elbow. (Fig. 36)

Raise body to an upright position, at the same time straightening knees. Also at the same time, lift curved right arm to a position near forehead, and lower left arm, with palm down, to front of left thigh; wrist is bent and fingers point north. Arms, body, and legs finish together. (Fig. 37)

Then as a separate movement, turn right hand to face palm upward, bending wrist.

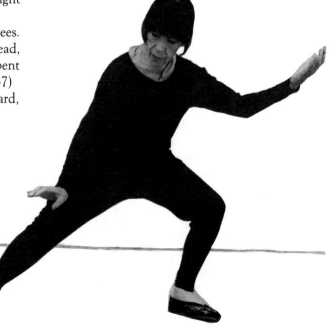

171

**Form 85. White Stork Flaps Its Wings**     *Pai Hao Liang Ch'ih*

Same as Form 7, Figures 38, 39, 40, 41, 42

Do not move right arm from its place near forehead for the next sequences.

Bend torso forward down, and at the same time, move left arm away from thigh so that it is perpendicular to floor. Palm faces floor. (Fig. 38)

Keep arms in same relative positions. Twist torso around to west, keeping body low. Arms move with body. Now left fingers point west; hand is at knee level. (Fig. 39)

Lift torso up erect, remaining turned toward west. At the same time bring straight left arm up to shoulder height. Left wrist is bent with palm west and fingers point upward. Head and torso are turned west; knees are straight; eyes look at left hand. (Fig. 40)

Turn torso to north. As you do this, bend left elbow and bring left hand to center of forehead with palm north so that left fingers point to right fingers; right palm is north. (Fig. 41)

Bend both knees, keeping back straight. At the same time, move both hands: bend wrists and turn hands so that palms face diagonally downward front; keep hands at forehead level. At the same time as hands move, press elbows diagonally forward so that right elbow points northeast and left elbow points northwest, both being at shoulder level. Make this movement with strength and hardness. Feel the contraction in the muscles of upper arms. This contrasts with the light and soft movements you have been using up to now. Feel as if you were holding or pressing the upper half of a ball between elbows and hands. Knees and hands move together (Fig. 42).

**Form 86. Brush Knee Twist Step**     *Lou Hsi Niu Pu*

Same as Form 8, Figures 43, 44

Keeping weight on right leg with its bent knee, shift right heel to east. This movement turns torso to face west, and at the same time, weight is released from left leg. Raise left heel off floor. As you move body and legs to west, turn right palm inward toward forehead, and turn left palm outward. Then circle left arm outward and downward, and move right arm down while left hand goes under right hand as right hand circles above left wrist. By this time, you are facing west. Both hands are ten inches away from chest: right palm faces south with fingers pointing west; elbow is down. Left wrist is bent with fingers north and palm west. (Fig. 172)

Moving left heel to west, place left heel in the Empty Step Space, with straight knee and flexed foot. Then transfer weight onto left leg, bending its knee and straightening right knee. Body slants forward west. As you step west, both arms move: move right arm to west in line with right shoulder, turning palm to face west with fingers pointing upward. At the same time, circle left arm with bent wrist downward and place left hand at front of left thigh. Palm faces floor with fingers pointing west. (Fig. 173)

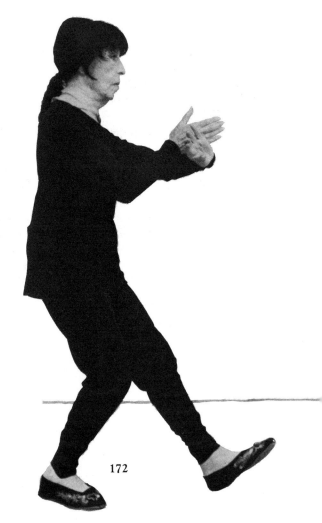

172

**Form 87. Hand Strums the Lute**  *Shou Hui P'i-P'a*

Same as Form 9, Figure 45

Shift weight back onto right leg bending right knee, and at the same time straighten left knee and flex foot. As legs move, both arms move: bring right arm inward, nine inches from face, keeping palm facing west with fingers pointing up. Move left hand upward and place fingertips at right pulse: left palm faces toward heart. Arms and legs move at the same time. (Fig. 174)

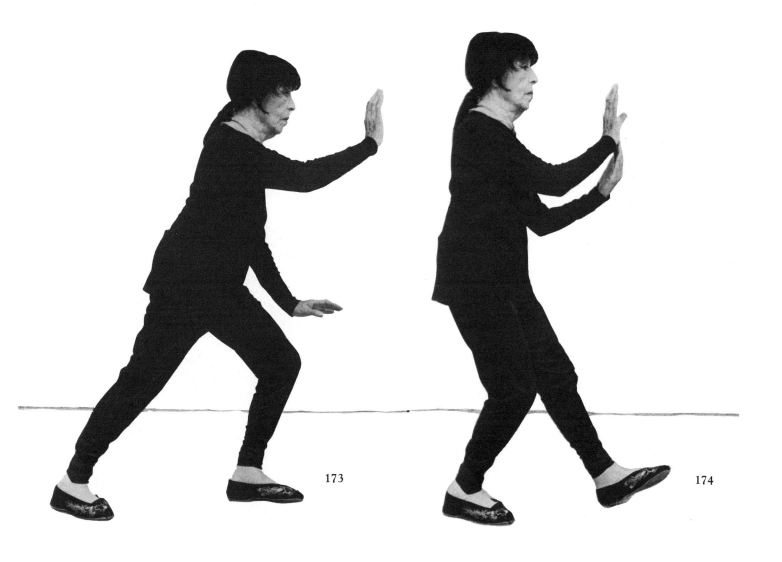

173

174

**Form 88. Needle at the Bottom of the Sea** *Hai Ti Chen*

Same as Form 26, Figure 77

Draw left foot, with loose ankle, to right foot, touching toes on floor. Weight is on right leg. At the same time, lower torso by bending more deeply on right knee and lean torso forward on a diagonal. Keep spine straight—do not curve back. On body and leg movement, start to move both arms: turning right palm south and left palm north, move right arm diagonally downward, with straight wrist, and gradually straighten right elbow. At the same time, move left palm close along right forearm to right inner elbow: left wrist bends gradually. Right arm is straight; left wrist and elbow are bent. Arms, legs, and body finish movements together. (Fig. 175)

**Form 89. Fan Through the Back** *Shan T'ung Pai*

Same as Form 27, Figures 78, 79, 80

Keep weight on right leg. Raise torso and direct it to northwest angle. At the same time, lift both arms, pointing right fingers up to northwest angle, at shoulder level. Left hand remains at right inner elbow.

Then place left foot in front of right, with its heel in line with right toes, turning left toes inward to point northwest. Straighten left knee. Right knee is close to left leg. Head looks northwest. (Fig. 78)

Shift weight onto left leg, bending left knee and straightening right knee. At the same time, begin to move both arms: slide (without touching) left fingers along right forearm toward northwest and draw right arm to right side. Left fingertips are at right palm when left knee is bent and right knee is straight. Left elbow is down. Right elbow is in line with right hand. (Fig. 79)

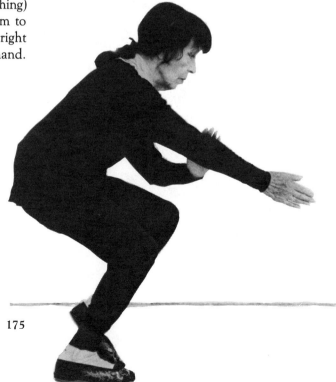

175

Keeping weight on left bent leg, move right heel slightly inward, making foot parallel to left. Then turn right toes outward to point northeast, bending right knee to equal that of left knee bend. You are now seated evenly on both legs, facing northeast. As you move right heel and toes, continue to move both arms: move left arm, which is shoulder high, to northwest with palm facing northwest and fingers up, and move bent right arm, shoulder high, to right side of head. Then turn right palm outward and up when arm gets into position behind right ear. Left arm is straight, right arm is curved. Eyes look at back of left hand. (Fig. 176)

**Form 90. Turn Body—Throw Fist**     *Fan Shien P'ieh Shen Ch'ui*
Same as Form 28, Figures 81, 82
Keeping weight on left leg with bent knee, move left toes inward slightly to northeast. Then move left heel outward to west, and on this heel movement straighten right knee. Keep right foot on floor. As left toes and heel move, upper torso is shifted to face northeast; head is now looking north. While you move left toes and heel, both arms move: circle left arm downward, fingertips inward, making hand into a fist, and place it near left hipbone, with fist-palm facing down. Circle right arm, fingertips inward, gradually making hand into a fist, then downward and inward to left hip. Place right fist above left with fist-palm down. Both fists arrive in position at the same time with movements of left heel. When fists meet, pull shoulders forward, moving elbows slightly forward. Use a hard force similar to Pressing the Ball. (Fig. 81) Left elbow is north, right elbow is east.

Move right toes to point east, shifting weight onto right leg, bending its knee, and straightening left kneee. Body slants forward east. At the same time, both arms move: move right fist up to east, chest high, with fist-palm facing east; wrist is bent. Move left fist, keeping it close behind right fist, gradually opening hand and spreading fingers wide apart; left is behind right fist. Wrist is bent: left palm faces right fist, with left fingers pointing upward. Both elbows are low. (Fig. 82)

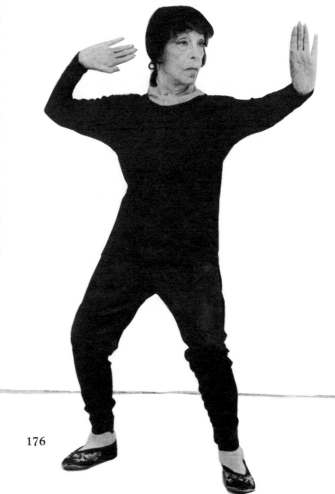

176

**Form 91. Step Up, Parry, and Punch**     *Chin Pu Pan Lan Ch'ui*

Shift weight back onto left leg bending knee, straightening right knee and flexing foot. At the same time, both hands move: turn left palm to face south and gradually place fingers together; turn right fist to face left palm. Draw right fist toward right hip, turning right fist-palm upward, elbow moving back to point west. Left arm goes shoulder high with straight wrist. (Fig. 177)

Shift weight forward onto right leg bending its knee, and straightening left knee. At the same time, move right fist forward east, and bend left wrist turning palm inward, fingertips south. Place right fist in front of left palm which is centered chest high. (Fig. 178) Draw left foot with loose ankle up to right foot.

**Form 92. Grasping the Bird's Tail**     *Lan Ch'ueh Wei*

Same as Form 30, Figures 25, 26, 27, 28

Circle left hand downward around right fist (keeping close to it) and place left fingertips at right pulse. Open right hand and point fingers to east. At the same time, step forward east on left foot bending left knee and straightening right knee. Body is on a slant forward east.

Shift weight back onto right leg, bending knee, straightening left knee, and flexing foot. At the same time, draw both arms inward toward body, chest high, keeping hands in same relationship. Elbows bend downward. Shift weight onto left leg, bending knee and straightening right leg. Draw right foot with loose ankle close to left foot; do not touch floor. At same time turn right palm up and left palm down; angle left hand so that it is at right angles to right hand. (Fig. 25 and Fig. 26 for hands)

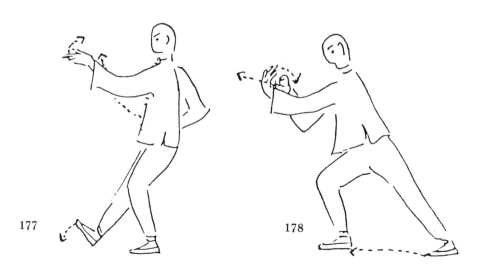

177          178

Then step right heel out to east in the Empty Step Space and transfer weight onto right leg, bending its knee and straightening left knee. Body is on a slant forward east. At the same stretch right arm to northeast, straightening right elbow. Keep left fingers at right pulse. (Fig. 27)

Circle both arms horizontally, shoulder high, from northeast to east, to southeast. When arms reach southeast, bend right elbow downward and bend right wrist so that palm faces upward. Both left and right fingers point southwest at the end of this horizontal circling. Left arm is adjusted to movement of right arm because left fingertips always remain near right pulse. (Fig. 27)

After circling arms to southeast, shift weight back onto left leg, bending its knee, and straighten right knee and flex foot. (Fig. 28)

Pivoting on right heel, turn right toes to northeast. At the same time, raise right arm with palm leading up, arc it over and down toward northeast, straightening arm as you do so. Stop in a position when right wrist is slightly above shoulder height.

As you are approaching this last position with right arm, put toes on floor bending right knee, placing weight on right leg and straightening left knee. Then bend right wrist and lower hand with fingers pointing downward, in Grasping position. Right arm remains in place while hand moves. Left fingers remain at right pulse. (Fig. 29)


**Form 93. The Single Whip**  *Tan Pien*
Same as Form 5, Figures 30, 31
Hold weight on right leg. Draw left foot with loose ankle close to right foot, not touching floor. Then move left leg to southwest diagonal in the Walking Step Space. Straighten left knee and place foot parallel to right foot. Body slants toward northeast. At the same time, move left arm down and in toward body chest high. As arm is moving, palm is up toward the face. Head moves from right to left side. Eyes look at left palm as it moves. (Fig. 179)

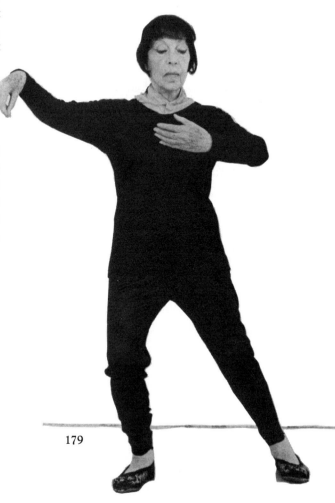

179

Turn left toes to point northwest. Bend left knee to equal that of right knee. Weight is even on both legs. Back is straight. Torso faces northwest. On movement of left toes, turn left hand to face northwest. Eyes look at back of left hand. (Fig. 180)

## SERIES VI

### Form 94. On Right—High Pat the Horse  *Kao T'an Ma*
Same as Form 34, Figures 93, 94

Keeping weight on right leg, move right toes inward slightly. Then move right heel outward to east and straighten left knee, keeping left foot on floor. This movement on right foot turns torso to west. At the same time as you move right foot, bend right elbow downward and raise right hand upward, opening hand; and then bring hand inward toward right shoulder with palm south. Left palm now faces north. (Fig. 93)

Weight remains on right leg with its bent knee. Draw left foot with loose ankle back and place it close to right foot; touch toes to floor. Back is straight. At the same time, both arms move: move left palm upward; draw left arm inward: left elbow goes to left side at hip height. Palm is up with straight wrist. Move right arm high with palm facing south; keep elbow high so that hand is at face level. Right elbow is bent at a right angle. Left palm is at the same vertical plane as right elbow. Arms are separated by width of body. (Fig. 94)

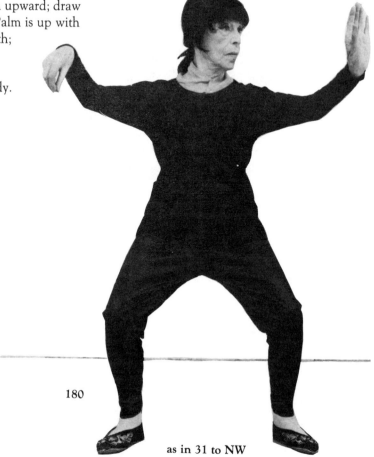

180

as in 31 to NW

### Form 95. Side—Face Palm   *P'i Mien Chang*

Place left heel forward west in the Empty Step Space; transfer weight onto left leg bending knee and straightening right knee. Body is on a slant forward west. At the same time both arms move: place right hand with palm downward at left armpit: elbow is high, level with hand. Move left arm forward west in line with left shoulder, turning palm to face west with fingers pointing upward. (Fig. 181)

### Form 96. Turn Body—Lotus Leg Cross   *Shih-Tzu Pai Lien Chiao*

Keep weight on left leg. Turn left toes inward to point north. At the same time, torso turns north and left arm moves with body: gradually straighten wrist, facing palm down, keeping it shoulder high. Do not move right arm. (Fig. 182)

Move right heel inward, bending right knee slightly. Then move left heel outward to west and straighten right knee; at the same time, torso and left arm move to northeast: move left arm, gradually bending elbow, at shoulder level in a horizontal circle, directing hand onto right shoulder, palm down. Do not move right arm. (Fig. 183)

Begin to draw right foot with loose ankle to left foot, and straighten left knee at same time; turn left palm upward raising it to head level. Torso faces east. (Fig. 184)

Draw right knee up and place foot with loose ankle near left knee. At the same time continue to move left arm outward to north, shoulder high, with palm north and fingers pointing up. (Fig. 185) Then move it in a horizontal circle at shoulder level toward east, gradually straightening wrist:

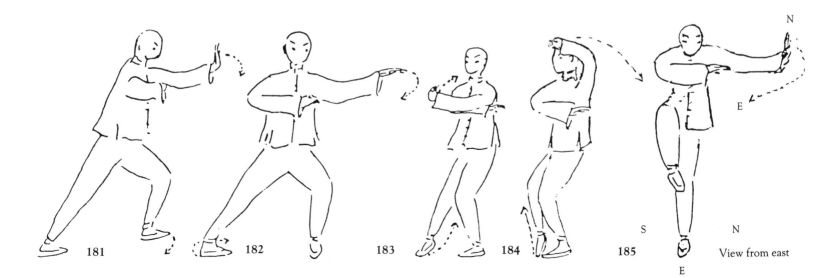

181   182   183   184   185   View from east

palm faces down. As arm circles toward east, extend and move right leg directly to east. Then, with foot flexed, touch left hand to right toes; bend body forward. Extended left hand and extended right leg meet at the same time. Do not move right arm. (Fig. 186)

### Form 97. Straight Center Punch    *Chih Tang Ch'ui*

Keep weight on left leg. Bend right knee and bring right leg back placing foot with loose ankle near left knee. At the same time, draw right elbow to right hip and make a fist of right hand, pulling right elbow back to west; turn right fist-palm upward at right hip. Left arm remains at left shoulder level: turn palm *south* with fingers toward east, and pull left arm inward, slightly bending elbow down. (Fig. 187)

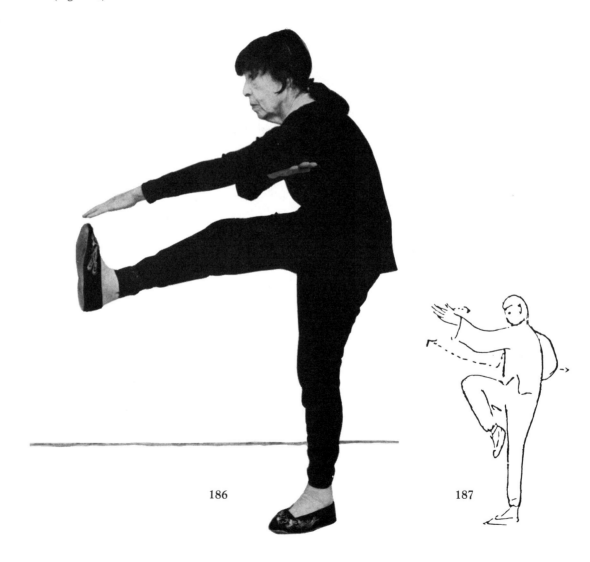

186                                                   187

Step forward east *quickly* on right foot; then *quickly* step forward on left foot, bending its knee and straightening right knee. Body is on a slant forward east. This is done extremely quickly—like a flash. As you step quickly on right, pull right fist back at right hip and push left arm slightly outward toward east, as if you were opening a bow to shoot an arrow.

As you step on left foot, punch right fist east, chest high. At the same time, move left palm to right inner elbow; wrist is bent and fingers point upward. Elbow is bent. This punch is done with hard force. Keep heel of right foot on floor. (Fig. 188)

### Form 98. Grasping the Bird's Tail     *Lan Ch'ueh Wei*

Same as Form 30, Figures 25, 26, 27, 28

Shift weight back onto right leg, bending its knee, straightening left knee, and flexing foot. At the same time, move left fingers to right pulse and open right hand keeping fingers pointing east. (Fig. 25 for arms)

Keep the relationship of hands the same; move both arms inward toward body to within 9 inches of chest, with both elbows bent downward and slightly out. Turn right palm up and left palm down. As you move hands, angle left hand so that it is at right angles to right wrist: now left elbow points north. At the same time as hands turn, shift weight forward onto left leg bending its knee and straightening right knee: body is on slant forward east. (Fig. 26 for arms only)

Then draw right foot with loose ankle close to left foot.

Place right heel forward east in the Empty Step Space, bending right knee and straightening left knee. Body slants forward at the same time as you step forward, stretching right arm to northeast with straight elbow. Keep left fingers at right wrist. (Fig. 27)

Circle both arms horizontally shoulder high, going from northeast, to east, to southeast. When arms reach southeast bend right elbow downward, bending right wrist so that palm faces upward. Turn right fingers to point to southwest. Left arm is adjusted to movement of right arm. Left fingers stay at right pulse (Fig. 28)

As you are bending arms from southeast, shift weight back onto left leg by bending left knee and straightening right knee and flexing foot. (Fig. 28)

Pivoting on right heel, turn toes to northeast. At the same time, raise right arm with palm leading up, head high; circle it over and down toward northeast, straightening arm as you do so, and stop in position when right wrist is slightly above shoulder height.

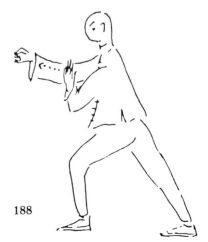

188

As you are approaching this last position with right arm, place right toes on floor, bend right knee, placing weight on right leg and straightening left knee. Then bend right wrist and lower hand, so that fingers point downward in grasping position: right arm remains in place while right hand moves. Left fingers remain near right pulse; left palm is toward your face. Left wrist is straight and arm is curved. (Fig. 189)

**Form 99. The Single Whip**   *Tan Pien*

Same as Form 5, Figures 30 and 31

Hold weight on right leg with its bent knee. Draw left foot with loose ankle close to right foot, not touching floor. Then move left leg backward to southwest diagonal in the Walking Step Space. Straighten left knee and place foot parallel to right foot: weight is on right, with body on a diagonal slant toward northeast. As left leg moves, move left arm, with palm toward your face, in a downward curve, in toward body, chest high. Eyes look at palm of left hand as it moves; do not tilt head. Head moves from right to left side. Right arm does not move. (Fig. 30)

Continue moving left arm up and outward toward northwest, and then pivoting on left heel, turn toes to point northwest. Place weight on left leg and bend knee to equal that of right knee. Now your weight is even on both legs. Back is straight and body is turned northwest. Turn left palm to face northwest as you move left toes. Both arms are at a little above shoulder level. Head is northwest and eyes look at back of left hand. (Fig. 190)

**Form 100. Snake Creeps Down**   *She Shen Hsia Shih*

Same as Form 79, Figures 157, 158, 159, 160

Turn left palm upward, as weight is shifting gradually to left leg, straightening right knee and lifting right heel off floor. As weight shifts move both arms: bend left elbow shoulder high bringing hand to head level, wrist bent and palm up; hand is vertically above elbow which is a right angle bend. Right arm moves after left hand has turned palm up: bending elbow shoulder high lift right hand up and bring it a little above forehead, palm up. Fingers of both hands point west and are twelve inches apart (Fig. 157). *Do not move arms* but *quickly* step right leg out to northeast on a diagonal, bending knee slightly and straightening left leg. Then move both hands with palms up around to south, then to southeast, then the right hand moves with palm up to northeast at head level, straightening elbow, while left hand with palm up moves to forehead. At the ending of the arm movements, turn right toes out to northeast. Torso remains northwest. (Fig. 158)

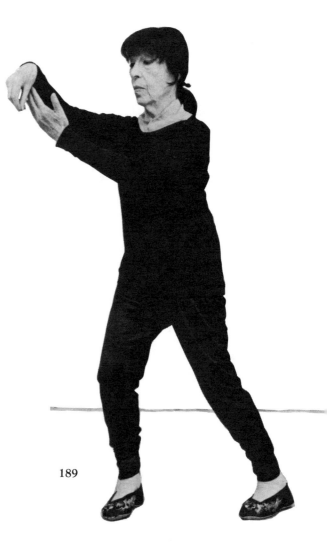

189

Keep weight on right leg. Turn left hand outward, then bend wrist so that fingers point north and palm east, all the while lowering arm to chest height, five inches away. Left elbow is on horizontal line with wrist. At same time, bend right wrist so that palm faces inward and fingers point diagonally down, moving hand in a southwest path to shoulder level, slightly in front of it. Right elbow is higher than hand. (Fig. 159)

Arms, torso and right knee bend moving together: Turn torso northwest and then bend it forward northwest. Move left hand, straightening wrist with fingers pointing diagonally downward northwest; right hand straightening wrist moves on a southwest path and stops at left elbow joint, palm inward. Both wrists are straight; head and torso are northwest. While all movement goes toward northwest, keep lowering the right knee-bend. The torso will therefore be weighted toward the right side, even though it is bending and leaning forward toward the left northwest direction. (Fig. 160)

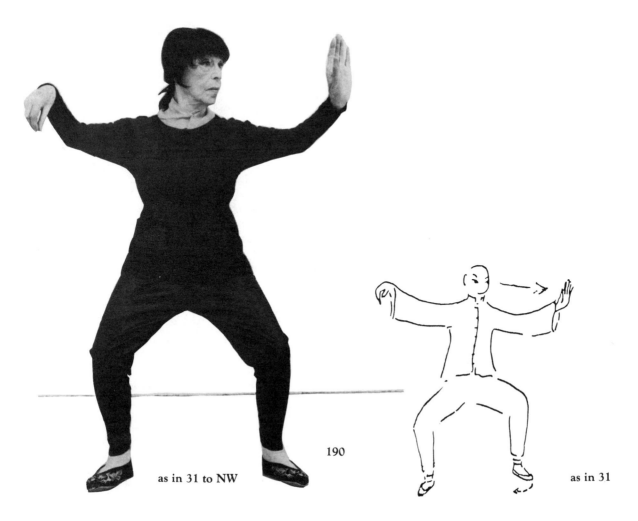

190

as in 31 to NW

as in 31

**Form 101. Step Up to Form Seven Stars** *Shang Pu Ch'i Hsing*

Shift weight onto left leg bending its knee. At the same time both arms move: start to raise left arm upward to left with fingers pointing to west, and move right arm vertically downward with fingers pointing to floor. Wrists are straight. (Fig. 161)

At the same time as arms are moving, turn right toes to point northwest straightening right knee. Then move left heel inward to make foot point west, weight is on left leg with its bent knee. The movements of right toes and left heel turn torso to face west. Body is on a slant forward west. While you shift toes and heel, complete the movements of arms: move left arm upward in line with left shoulder, with palm north and fingers west; and move right arm downward vertically at right side, with palm inward toward body and fingers pointing downward. (Fig. 162)

Keep weight on left leg with its bent knee and with torso on a slant forward west. Draw right foot with loose ankle close to left foot. Then move right leg to west. Straighten knee and place foot flat on floor, toeing-in slightly. At the same time, arms move: lower left arm and hand chest high; bring right arm up to west with palm south, and place right hand near left hand so that left thumb is at center of right palm. At the same time, when right hand reaches this position, move both wrists (without moving arms out of place) bend left hand downward diagonally and spread fingers wide apart; bend right hand upward diagonally and spread fingers wide apart. (Fig. 191)

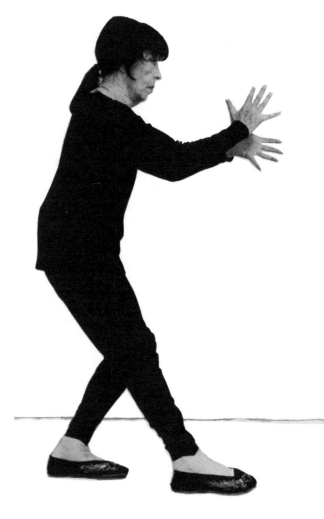

191

## Form 102. Retreat Step and Ride the Tiger *T'ui Pu K'ua Hu*

Keep weight on left leg with its bent knee. Bring right foot with loose ankle back near left foot. At the same time, both hands move: passing each other, right hand goes downward and left hand upward over right wrist. As hands are moving, draw fingers of each hand close together, so that hands are in their usual form, with palm curved and fingers close. Wrists are diagonally crossed with hands facing the diagonals.

Keep weight on left with its bent knee. Place right leg backward to east in the Walking Step Space, straightening right knee. At the same time as leg moves, lower torso down west, and bring both arms down to a perpendicular knee level. Hands are crossed at wrists. (Fig. 192)

Move right toes to northeast and move bent-over torso to north, arms moving with torso. Keep moving torso while right toes move northeast. Bend right knee, straightening left knee at the same time as torso moves northeast. Arms are now near right knee. (Fig. 193)

Turn left toes to north and at the same time, bend both wrists so that fingers of both hands point east: right palm faces floor and left palm faces up. Fold left fingers over left thumb as wrists bend. (Fig. 194)

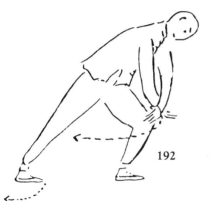
192

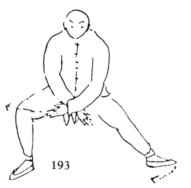
193

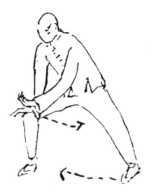
194

NE

138     Separate arms at the same time: right goes up toward east with wrist bent so that fingers point upward. Left arm goes toward west with bent wrist leading and fingers pointing downward. At the same time, move left leg with loose ankle close to right foot. (Fig. 195)

Bring left leg with bent knee up forward to northeast and then begin to straighten right knee. Begin to lift torso to an upright position. At the same time, both arms continue to move: right goes up to east and left goes up to west, until they reach positions a little higher than shoulder level. Head is northeast, hips are straight and even; shoulders are straight and even. Torso faces north. Left leg is high and is pulled over to northeast with foot pointed inward. Right palm faces east. Left hand is in grasping position toward west. Left leg, torso, and arms arrive in position at the same time. (Fig. 196)

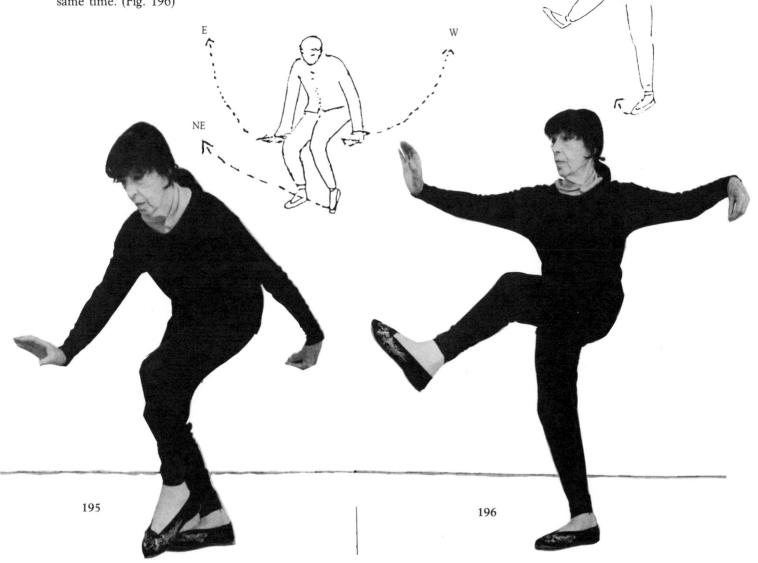

195

196

# Form 103. Turn Around and Swing Leg (Lotus Swing)

*Chuan Shen Pai Lien*

Lower left elbow downward and draw left hand toward left shoulder; at the same time, raise hand up with palm to north.

Pivot on right heel, placing toes east. This movement turns body to face east. Right arm shoulder high extends to east, palm is east. Do not move left leg out of position on pivot. (Fig. 197)

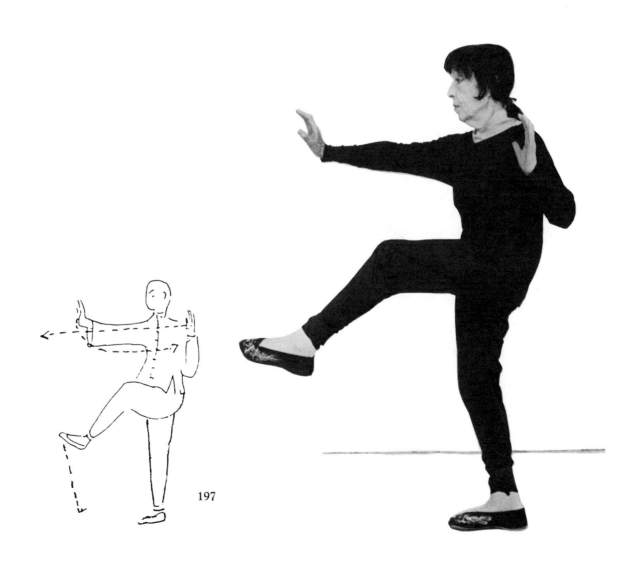

197

140    Keep weight on right leg. Bend more deeply on right knee, lowering body and place left foot on floor to east with toes inward and with straight knee. At the same time, place right hand with palm down at left armpit and extend left arm to east in line with left shoulder: palm is east. (Fig. 199) Sequence shown in Figure 198.

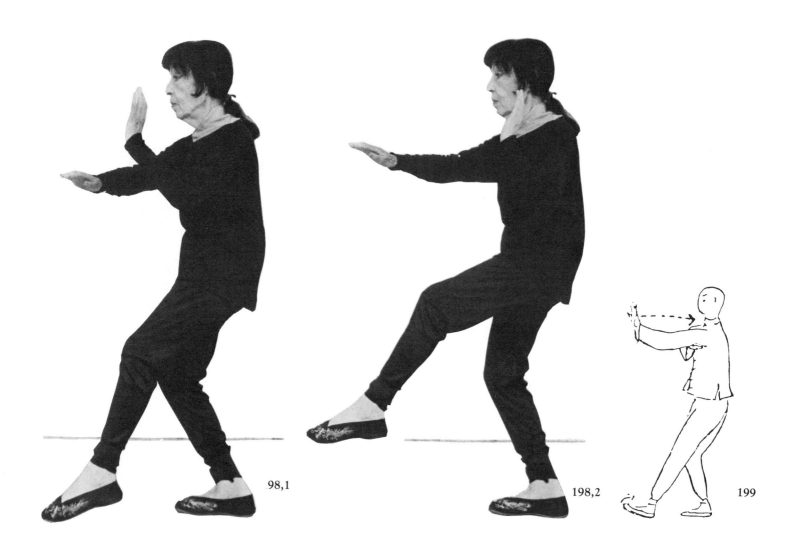

98,1

198,2

199

(1) Turn left toes inward to southeast and straighten left wrist moving palm down. (2) Bend left knee, straightening right, lean toward southeast, and continue to move left arm shoulder high to south. (Fig. 200) (3) Curve left arm going on a slight downward path and approach right elbow while right heel moves inward. (4) Turning torso to southwest, put left hand under right armpit and place right hand above left shoulder. (5) Pivot left heel outward—which moves torso to west, and lift right hand to forehead, palm out. Left arm does not move; right toes stay on floor. (Fig. 201)

Lift right leg and bring foot with loose ankle near left knee: right knee points west and right foot is toed in. At the same time as leg lifts, both arms move: move right arm out to north shoulder high with palm facing north and fingers up. Move left arm up curved, above head, with palm up. (Fig. 202) Then move left arm to south; palm south.

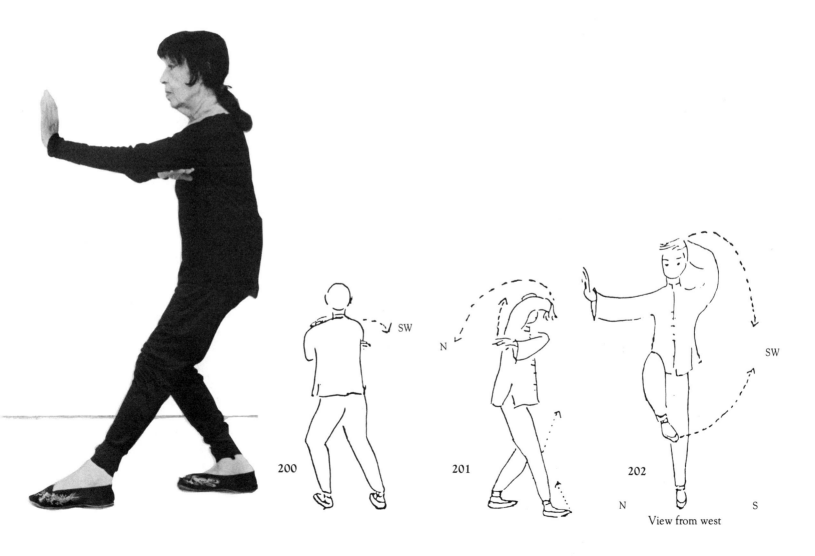

200

201

202

View from west

Swing-circle right leg very *quickly*: swing it to southwest pointing toe and then to west flexing foot. (Fig. 203, 204)

Quickly place foot down in the Walking Step Space west. Body slants forward west. (Fig. 205)

For Figures 203 and 204 arms must move quickly. For Figure 203 slap-strike right foot on its inner side with left palm as foot swings to southwest. For Figure 204 slap-strike right foot on its outer side with right palm as right foot swings to west. Bend body down and toward west in order to strike foot. The tempo is extremely fast. (Fig. 206)

After striking foot with left hand, bring arm up curved in front of forehead, with palm up. After right hand strikes, bring right arm up toward northwest with palm up and fingers pointing northwest. The arms go into place as right leg goes into Walking Step Space with bent knee: left knee straightens. Hands are about twelve inches apart. Left arm is curved and right is straight. (Fig. 205)

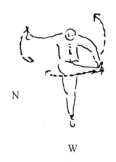

N

W

View from west

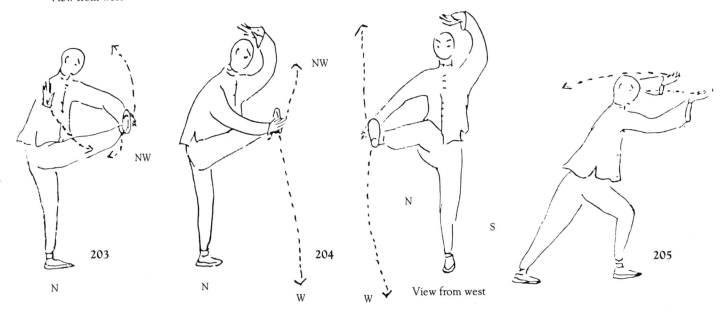

203 N

204 N W

N S W View from west

205

## Form 104. Curve Bow Shoot Tiger    *Wan Kung She Hu*

Move arms together from northwest angle. Bend both elbows bringing hands downward toward forehead; wrists will bend; palms are upturned. Keep hands twelve inches apart. From forehead level, arc hands toward southeast downward, arriving at waist height; left elbow is near body at side and right hand is at left hip slightly in front; finger-tips point southeast. Continue the movement by moving hands in front at abdomen level; wrists and elbows straighten and palms lead the upward curve toward the northwest. Right arm is head high; left is eye high; both palms are north. Body and legs do not move. (Figures 206-207 and 208)

Do not move legs, body, or head. Move both arms at the same time: bend left elbow downward and draw hand, making a fist of it, to left shoulder: fist-palm faces north; wrist is bent so that knuckes of fist are directed west. Bend right elbow, keeping it high, pointing to north, and draw hand, making a fist of it, eye high, to side of face. Wrist is bent so that fist-palm faces north and knuckles point west. (Fig. 209)

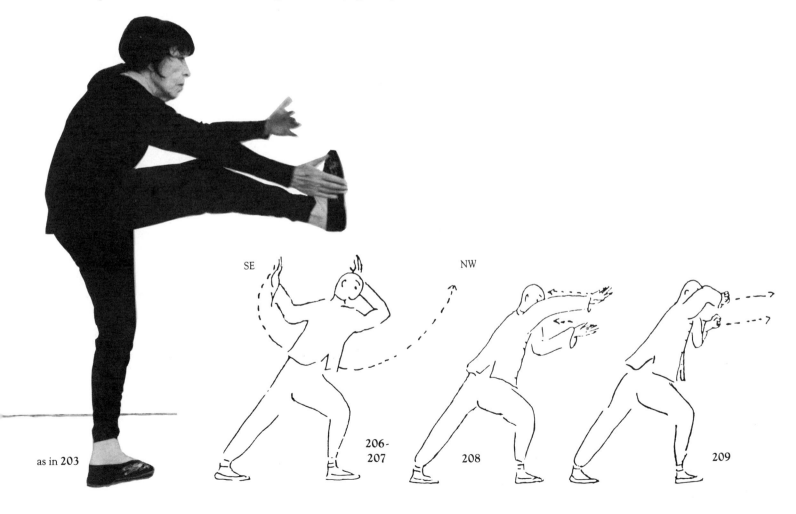

as in 203

SE    NW

206-
207     208     209

Do not move legs, head, or body. Move both arms outward to west, each on its own level: right is eye high and left is shoulder high. Fist-palms remain facing north. Fists stop in the same vertical plane, 15 inches from body with right arm curved high and left arm angled low. (Fig. 210)

### Form 105. On Right—High Pat the Horse    *Kao T'an Ma*

Similar to Form 34, Figure 94)

Shift weight back onto left leg, bending knee and straightening right knee. Lower torso forward and then twist torso to face southwest. Keep right foot on floor; keep head facing west. At the same time both arms move: gradually opening both fists, place right hand outward and left hand inward. Bring right hand under left arm and place right hand with palm facing down at left armpit. Left arms circles over right, elbow bends with hand on a diagonal toward floor, abdomen high. Both wrists are straight: right elbow points west and left elbow points south. Head looks west (Fig. 211)

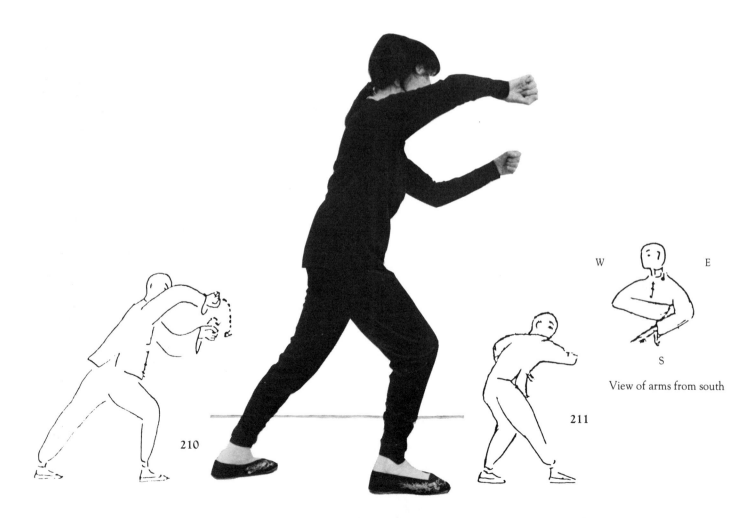

210

211

View of arms from south

Then lean torso, straighten left leg and bend right knee. Body is southwest. Turn torso to face west with weight forward on right leg, bending its knee, and straighten left knee. Draw left foot with loose ankle close to right foot and place left toes on floor near right foot. At the same time, circle right arm toward west as torso turns to face west. Move right arm high so that hand faces south at head level. Move left elbow to left hip, turning palm up. Both wrists are straight. Left palm and right elbow are on same level; arms are separated by width of body. (Fig. 94)

**Form 106. Side Face Fist—and Turn Body**   *P'i Mien Ch'üan Chuan Shen*
Same as Form 95, Figure 181
Place left heel forward west in the Empty Step Space; transfer weight onto left leg bending knee and straightening right knee. Body is on a slant forward west. At the same time both arms move: place right hand, making it into a fist, (this differs from Form 95) at left armpit: fist-palm faces down and elbow is high. Move left arm forward west in line with left shoulder, turn palm to west with fingers pointing up. (Fig. 181 with right *fist* instead of open hand)

WARRIOR FORM      *Wu Shih*
Keep weight on left leg with its bent knee. Turn left toes inward. Torso turns north and left arm moves with body: gradually straighten wrist and make a fist with fist-palm facing floor. Do not move right arm. (Fig. 182, with fists instead of open hands)

Move right heel inward, bending right knee slightly. Left arm moves in a horizontal circle on a slight downward path with fist approaching right armpit. (Fig. 212)

*Quickly* move left fist under right arm to right armpit; then in quick sequence remove right fist from left armpit making it go in front of left arm. (Fig. 213) Torso moves northeast slowly.

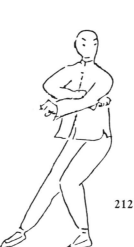

212

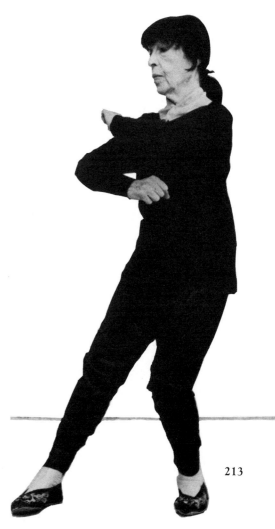

213

Next in slow succession move left fist in front of left shoulder and right fist in front of right shoulder bringing elbows close to body while moving left heel to west and turning torso to east. Turn both fists east and then slowly open hands to face east; elbows point downward.

While both hands are opening, flex right foot, straightening right knee. Weight is on left leg with its bent knee. (Fig. 214)

### Form 107. Carry Tiger To Mountain    *Pao Hu Kuei Shan*

Reverse of Form 14, Figures 52, 53

Shift weight onto right leg forward east, bending right knee and straightening left. At the same time, push both hands, which face east, forward shoulder high to east, each arm in line with its shoulder. Wrists are shoulder high; fingers point upward; body slants forward east. (Fig. 215)

Keep weight on right leg with its bent knee. Bend torso forward and down moving arms at the same time. Arms are lowered so that palms face floor at knee level. Arms are perpendicular to floor. (Fig. 216)

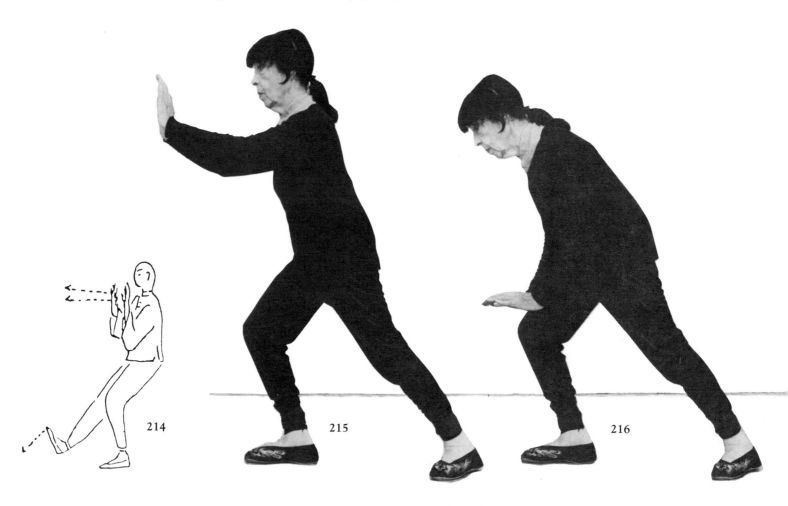

214

215

216

# Form 108. Closing Form of T'ai-Chi Ch'üan   *He T'ai Chi*

First move torso northeast and then turn left toes to north. Shift weight onto left leg bending its knee and straighten right knee. With these movements move torso to north, still remaining bent over. As you move left toes, move left arm to left side of left leg, with palm facing floor and fingers to west. Right hand remains at right side with palm facing floor and fingers to east. (Fig. 217)

Lift torso up to an upright position and with it bring both arms up sideways to shoulder height. As arms move upward, gradually straighten wrists, and turn right toes north. (Fig. 218)

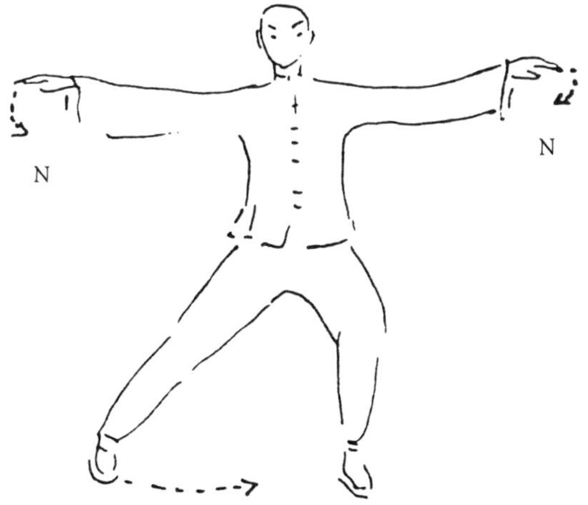

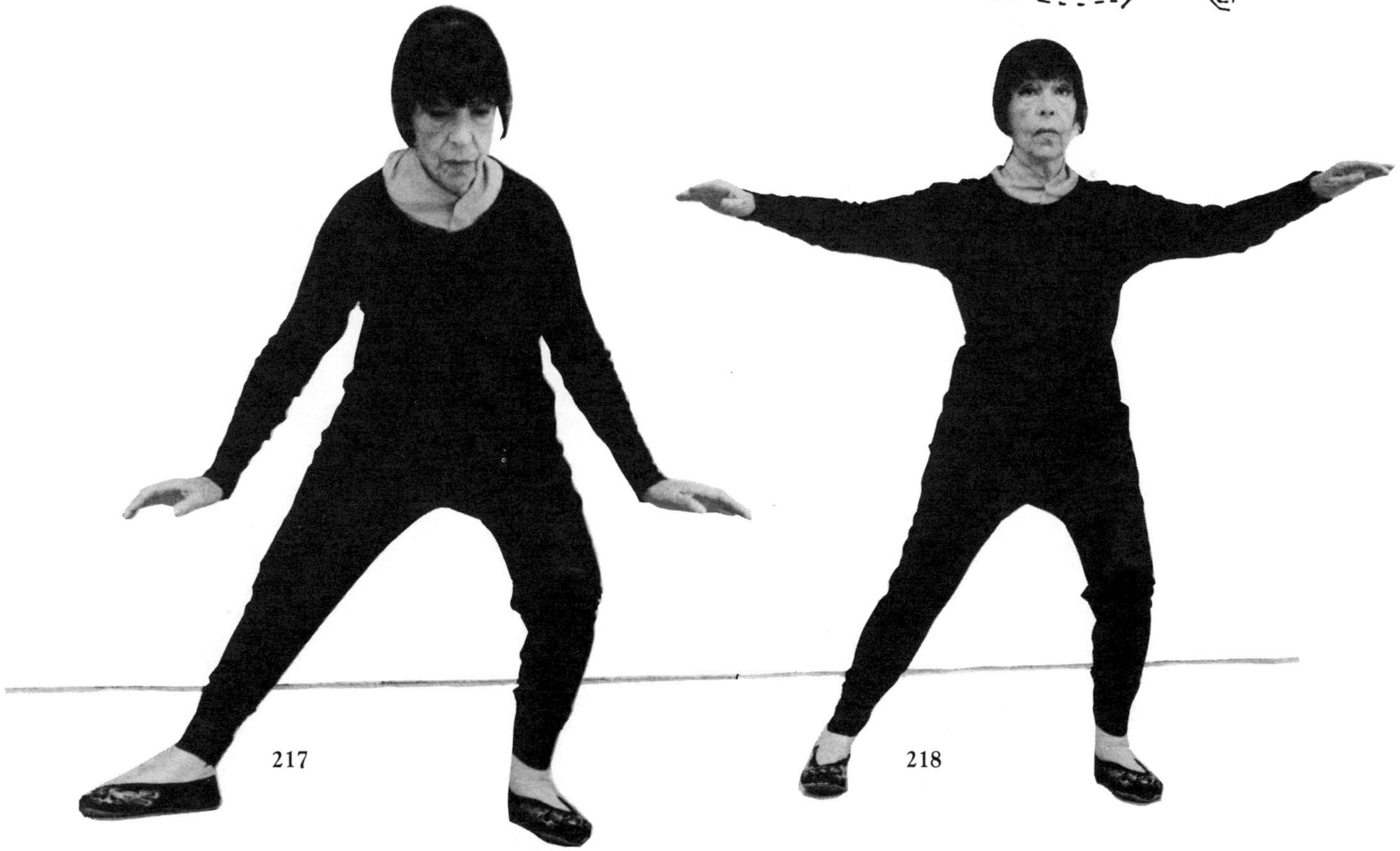

217

218

148 Keep weight on left leg with its bent knee. Move both arms forward at shoulder height to north: hands face floor; wrists are straight; arms are shoulder width apart. At the same time, move right foot and place it parallel to and apart from left foot in your basic stance. Both knees are equally bent. Back is straight. (Fig. 219)

Keeping arms in their forward parallel position shoulder high, gradually straighten knees. (Fig. 220)

Then, lower both arms to sides of thighs, right to right side, and left to left side. Palms face south and wrists are straight. You are now in exactly the same form and position with which you started t'ai-chi ch'üan. Your feet should be in exactly the same place where they were in the Beginning Form. (Fig. 221)

When you finish the entire exercise, remain standing quietly in position, holding the last posture. Release from this position when you "feel" like moving out of it.

This exercise is to be done on the left side, too. When you are proficient and perform the exercise in even tempo, flowingly and continuously, then you may learn it on the reverse side. To study it in this way will augment your knowlege of the subtle details, sharpen your concentration, and perfect your balance and skill. When you perform it relatively well, to increase your interest further you should try to do it very quickly, within ten minutes.

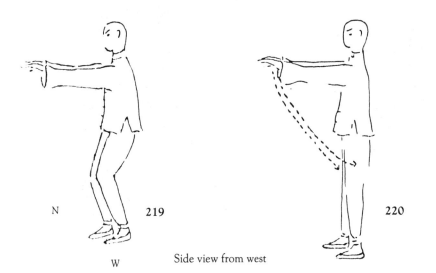

N        219                    220

W        Side view from west

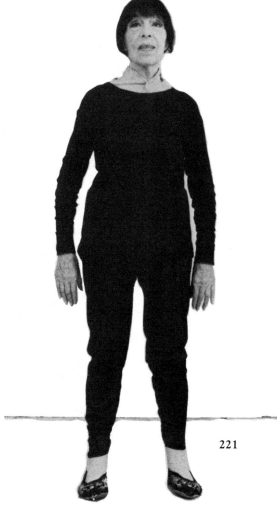

221

FORM 108

*Chang San-Feng's theories were documented and augmented by Wang*
*Chung-Yüeh (Ming Dynasty, circa fifteenth century). Following are excerpts from*
*his book and two other documents attributed to this period translated for me by*
*Koo Hsien-Liang, Hubert Wang, and Sally Ch'eng.*

1. T'AI-CHI CH'ÜAN LUN: T'ai-Chi Ch'üan Discourse.

T'ai-chi is infinity, the absolute; it creates from "no limit." It contains
dynamic and static movement; it is the mother of yin and yang, of everything
male and female. It is the root of motion, which is division, and of stillness,
which is union. It must neither be overdone nor underdone—it must be
exact. . . Comprehension comes from growing understanding plus effort
and this leads one gradually to full enlightenment. Unless one pursues
this exercise long enough one cannot hope to understand fully. . . .
Be open-minded (receptive-void) and concentrate on the top of the
head, with Ch'i marshaled in the abdomen. Tip in neither direction and
be "as if suddenly hiding, suddenly appearing." If left side is weighted it is
then ready to change to void (*Hsü*); if right side is weighted (*Shih*), then it
is ready to change to void. . . . When one looks from below upward at a
t'ai-chi ch'üan master, he appears to be lofty. The longer you look, the
loftier he appears. When you look at him from above downward, he looks
more "deep". . . . A feather cannot be added, nor a fly land without effecting
a change (in balance). . . . When a master stands he is in perfect balance
and moves as a carriage wheel does. . . . If one doesn't progress, it is probably
one's own fault because of bad habits. . . . One must know yin and yang;
yin does not leave yang and yang does not leave yin; they mutually help
each other. . . . Thus it is that comprehension (understanding plus effort)
leads to skill. By quietly studying and analyzing, one gradually learns to
do—at the bidding of the mind. Theoretically one should forget oneself
and learn from others. The prevailing mistake is to seek things which one
is not yet equipped to learn. By making even a tiny mistake, one can go
wrong by a thousand miles. This leads dangerously to endless blunders.
Beginners would do well to bear this in mind and should study
discriminatingly.

2. SHIH-SAN SHIH KO: Song of the Thirteen Kinetic Movements (ward
off slantingly upward, pushing, pressing forward or squeezing, pushing
downward, gathering, twisting, elbowing, leaning, stepping forward, stepping
backward, looking right, looking left, and being centered). Never neglect
any of the thirteen kinetic changes.
All important thought should be aimed at the vital junctures. You must
be attentive to the slightest change from *Hsü* (empty) to *Shih* (solid). . . . A

movement has its seeds in the state of stillness before it is seen . . . . In every movement one must analyze the hidden meaning. When well-done all appears effortless. Pay attention to the waist at all times. With abdomen loose and light, Ch'i can move (be in full swing). If coccyx is properly centered, the "spirit" rises from the top of the head. Body is so light that only head matters. If you pay attention to the push and pull, expansion-contraction, bend and stretch, open and close, you will then have full freedom and you can do anything you like. (Beginners best be guided by oral teaching.) Work incessantly and skill will take care of itself. What is meant by making good use of the body? The answer is the mind wills and the body obeys (guiding spirit-mind is the master and the body—bones and flesh—is the servant). Think what the final purpose is—that one will never grow old (spring will be eternal) . . . . If you do not search in this direction, it will be a sheer waste of effort and that would be such a pity!

3. SHIH-SAN SHIH HSING KUNG HSIN CHIEH: Treatise on the Thirteen Kinetic Movements As They Relate to Mental Comprehension.

Calmness is of decisive importance . . . . there will be perfect spontaneity only when everything is done according to the dictates of the mind. There will be no danger of being heavy and clumsy, or of not attaining lightness (at top of head) if the spirit co-operates.

Facility of action comes from change of movements from *Hsü* to *Shih* (from void to solid). Even when exerting effort one must be calm and appear effortless. One must concentrate and aim at one direction. The entire body must be loose, straight, comfortable, peaceful, quiet, centered . . . . One must be prepared to face any change in the eight directions . . . . Motion should be like refined steel. The form is like that of a hawk about to seize a rabbit; the spirit is like that of a cat about to catch a mouse. The quietness is like that of a mountain range; movement is agile, like a river.

Storing up energy is like that of an open bow; letting go (of effort-energy) is like that of letting the arrow go. Seek straightness in a curve. Store up energy before using it. Strength comes from the spine; steps follow body changes. Getting ready is as important as doing. It has continuity, though it has "broken movement." Like a pleat which folds in on itself and continues to the next one with rhythm and order, so the movement goes forward and back with rhythm and order and continuity. There must be changes, alterations, and variety. Only when one knows how to be "soft" can one be properly strong. Learn to breathe well and then you will have alacrity-alertness-speed. Ch'i must be cultivated without hindrance, as a result of which you will be able to do anything. Stamina is stored up, is saved, by moving in curves. The mind gives the orders (is in command); the breath is the banner; the waist is the leader (the hinge, the axis).

First learn to stretch and expand; then learn to contract and condense . . . . Then it will be possible to be perfectly integrated (be a master).

First conceive in the mind; then express in the body. Keep abdomen loose; breath permeates bones; give spirit free rein and the body will be calm. Be attentive all the time. Deeply remember: one single movement suffices to effect the whole body movement; there is no isolated quiet without enveloping the whole being . . . . Inside, one is firm, and outside, one shows peacefulness. The even pace is like that of a cat walking. The strength exerted is like that of pulling silk. One's attention is on the spirit, not on the breath . . . . too much preoccupation with breath makes one clumsy . . . . The appearance of "lack of breath" is real strength . . . .

*Authors of the special Chinese books on t'ai-chi ch'üan (to whom I referred, as translated for me by Hubert Wang and Koo Hsien-Liang) are: Wu Chien Ch'üan and Ma Yüeh-Liang, Tung Ying-Chieh, Ts'ai Ho Peng (a compilation), Wu T'u Nan, Ch'ang Ch'un, Hsu Chih-Yi, Dr. Ch'ü Mien-Yu.*

## ASPECTS OF SELF-AWARENESS

### AT THE BEGINNING — Becoming Still

At attention, light and easy,
   emptied of irrelevancies,
Full awareness of one's self.
Quietly alert, to sense
The moment before moving
   into space and form.

### DURING ACTION — Moving Intrinsically

Differentiating subtleties
   link in constant flow;
Multi-units balance instantly,
Body-mind in unison,
Centering magnetically
   on every passing change.

### AT THE ENDING — Being Still

All is one, lightly soaring
   yet contained,
Filled with something
Other than before —
The presence of a tranquil present —
   serene, secure.

### AFTER COMPLETION — Being Composed

Feeling calm contentment
   emptied of dilemmas,
Moving casually away
To normal functioning,
Clear-mindedly
   with energies enriched.

# Part Three:

*Interpretation*

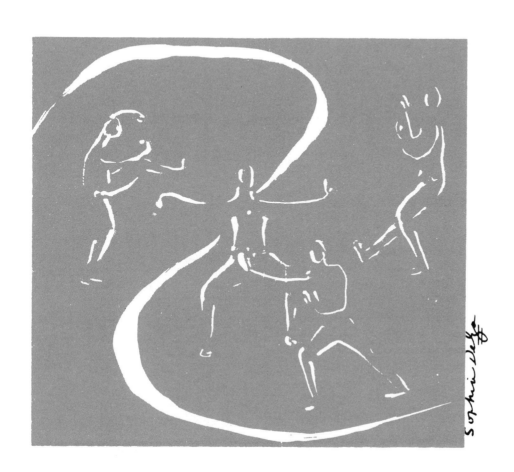

A world of movement, form, and structured action designed to achieve a state of heart-mind body harmony, t'ai-chi ch'üan can be said to be philosophically based and physiologically directed. With equal validity it can be conceived as being physically based and philosophically directed. Both are intrinsic concepts which balance each other since Meaning and Method cannot be separated by a hair's breadth.

Meaning is a composite of t'ai-chi ch'üan's goal and many faceted aims of which patience and attention, perception and insight, awareness and calmness are component parts, all generated in the process of experiencing the Method. These deeply-related qualities fuse harmoniously, resulting in the development of a high state of consciousness. This, as essence, is *one* dimensional, combining all interrelated, interacting aspects into a single-minded entity.

The substance of the Method, the exercising-system, is concerned with the organic laws of the Body, the activity of the Mind, and the significance of the Structure. These three are all interrelated on a multi-dimensional scale which includes concentration and coordination, form and design-pattern changes, movement in space-time relationships, balance and the accuracy of weight changes. All are uniquely organized in the action at every fraction of a second and are integrated in spirit to become and be the heart of the Meaning.

## I. Dimensions of Meaning

In the Sung Dynasty (960-1279) Chang San-Feng, designated as the Father of t'ai-chi ch'üan, was inspired to create a physical-mental Method, a conscious way, a systematized structure of movement and form, from which man could develop to a high state of self-knowledge; from which latent potentialities existing within him could be easily and subtly awakened. Tranquility, fundamental to such an ideal, would always be present, whether one was in a state of quiet or in a state of activity.

After thirty years of 'self' exploration, with mind-body relationship at its core, Chang San-Feng succeeded in giving a concrete structure to his philosophical and spiritual concepts—he had created an objective exercise-method, a universe of form and structure that would arouse in the heart-mind of the practitioner the 'Ultimate' Meaning—the essence of which had been his inspiration.

From the heart of the inner Meaning (the goal), the Method had come to fruition (1) with a technique that considered man's total being—

in the personal terms of body, mind, emotional and spiritual harmony and (2) with an objectively-designed, styled structure incorporating the universality of space-time, form-change, and the dynamic relationship of function to energy. These elements were minutely structured according to the physiological laws of nature to be harmoniously balanced at all times.

Chang's creation was a "Grand Universe of Structure": a mind-body exercise consisting of the T'ai-chi and a ch'üan. T'ai-chi represents the concept of the eternally moving interplay of the cosmic forces, termed yin and yang, complementary in nature, each necessary for the existence of the other. When they are in balance, equanimity results. The ch'üan is the body-action technique, a multiple process functioning according to the principle of the T'ai-chi where moving structure is in continuous succession and in natural harmony.

All aspects—physical, mental, emotional—are directed to develop complete health, and to enable man to function with skill in a multitude of situations with calmness and equanimity, with the far-reaching aim of attaining such profound awareness as to become a 'conscious' being.

The ch'üan forms and the T'ai-chi process (in immense variety) integrate in terms of the abstractions of space-time, gravitational force, and action-stillness, functioning in unity at every moment.

As T'ai-chi represents the fact that matter is in constant motion, so t'ai-chi ch'üan in a miniature way, mirrors the universal continuity of change with alternating flow of yin and yang and includes, along with the dynamics of lightness and strength, the intrinsic use of energy, and the proportion of space-form, the directional changes as well as the body's physicality of joint and muscle-related action.

Composite yin-yang activity renders the ch'üan impervious to excessive and false expenditure of one's physical as well as emotional resources. Correct action is regulated by the significant structure, the 'bones and flesh', as the Chinese say, of the Method.

The original creative source—that of "The Ultimate Meaning", had given life to the multiform Method. The Method arouses, evokes, inspires all shades of the purposeful Meaning at every stage and phase of the action and the structure. The Method is transmuted into Meaning. Chang San-Feng's philosophical, spiritual, and physical "Meaning", having given rise to the "Means," is now reborn by means of the Method. The synthesis of 'means and end' are the warp and woof of t'ai-chi ch'üan.

T'ai-chi ch'üan exists in and *is* its "Grand Universe" of significant structure, making Meaning and Method entities to be measured side by side as a unity.

To speak of a complete state of health is to presuppose physical and emotional-mental balance. Such balance can be called equanimity, free from negative emotions and anxiety. Each individual state—of ease, of calmness, of concentration—leads to another level of experience, that of consciousness and of equilibrium-tranquility (to repeat a quotation from the *I-Ching*—Chinese Book of Changes): "Tranquility is a kind of vigilant attention. It is when tranquility is perfect that the human faculties can display all their resources because (then) they are enlightened by reason and sustained by knowledge."

Such a peak of Meaning and experience can be compared to the flower that appears in its full glory after the plant has been growing well for some time. The growth and the gradually developing facets of coordination, attention, awareness, patience, and perception evolving from the activity of the exercise become a unity of 'oneness,' greater than the individual elements, unique and different. . .a feeling of being one with one's self, and with consciousness heightened. What one senses at the ending of the exercise when one is standing and holding still, is that:

All is one, lightly soaring,
  yet contained,
Filled with something,
  other than before—
The presence of a tranquil present—
  serene, secure.

This desirable state of being does not evaporate when t'ai-chi ch'üan ends and one returns to one's every day work-way. One important meaning of 'Meaning' is the possessing and retaining of a balanced condition of mind and body in any situation, even the most provocative— to have patience with oneself and others at all times; to be attentive and profoundly perceptive; and to be comfortably at ease—in short, to be a calm and conscious person.

After "learning" the t'ai-chi ch'üan Exercise, the state of mind is this:

Feeling calm contentment
  emptied of dilemmas,
Moving casually away
To normal functioning,
Clear-mindedly
  with energies enriched.

## II. Dimensions of Method

The immense range of the complex Method can be divided into several categories. But it must be kept in mind that they never function separately in the exercise, neither physically nor mentally.

The dimensions of the Method can be distinguished as (1) the way of the body; (2) the way of the mind; (3) the way of the structure. These overlap, interrelate, and penetrate each other; each way reflects some aspect of another way. At any given moment of action, body, mind, and structure blend as do the sounds made by several musical instruments played at the same time.

The unity of the Method's dimensions comes from the impeccable balance of all "ingredients": the physiological laws of body behavior, the ever-present attentive mind, and the unfailing balanced nature of the structure-organization without which there is no ch'uan.

Mental-physical control, patience, endurance, calmness, and coordination in integrating form and movement are substantial facets embedded in all three dimensions. Richly interwoven are form, tempo, space-direction, shape, dynamics, flow, continuity, balance—all precisely proportioned at each instant of action to awaken and produce the composite Meaning.

Because of the balanced nature of the complete entity, the relationship of each single part to the others can naively be taken for granted. But the understanding of how it all 'works' and the conscientious application of such knowledge increases the awareness of the harmonious whole and deepens experience of the unity of Meaning and Method.

## CHAPTER 7

## I. Way of the Body: Quiet Strength

The essential quality is the way of holding the body, with dignity, assurance and alertness. Dignity arises from the awareness of how the body itself behaves intrinsically — not from an extraneous thought of "wanting" it to be so. Assurance comes from the natural relationship of dynamic energy and movement, which is mentally perceived and controlled. Attention centered on the action is alertness. This composite way of holding the body coexists with the activity and is sustained by the way of the structure (page 164).

The correctly aligned physical body requires the spine be straight with coccyx 'tucked' under, so that the buttocks do not protrude "like a mountain top", (as the Chinese say); that the head be held "as if suspended from the heavens by a silken thread" (Chinese version). The shoulders are low and held without effort. The torso is natural, not arched, nor hollowed in, which would throw the shoulders forward. The pelvis-trunk section is firm as are the legs and feet. Hips and shoulders are aligned vertically. This stance, the normal position for everyone, anywhere, permits the body to move with ease and flexibility at all times,

The technique of movement is soft-intrinsic (page 18), position and form determining the amount of effort expended by muscles and joints, without emotional or intellectual interference. There is, therefore, no strained pressure in maintaining the continuous flow of movement as the patterns pass from one part of the body to the other. With no outlay of extraneous force, all designed positions are in physical equilibrium, so that every moment of the action is felt to be light and evenly balanced as if on a scale.

This sensation of lightness, a unique element ever present in this exercise, is a result of both the intrinsic dynamic changes and the impeccable proportions of physical forms in terms of space and time, position and placement.

All the component parts of the exercise are put into harmony by the organic relationship of the different parts of the body's moving structure. The way the body acts reveals certain characteristics that seem to reflect and express some of the goals to be achieved, such as calmness, patience, stillness and equilibrium.

Each part, each segment of the body possesses an interesting 'completeness', a quality which reflects and describes the way it functions. All together the variegated attributes make a distinctive 'landscape' of the self, physically and psychologically.

Individualized, the following attributes can be considered basic to each designated part in a finely organized body, in action or repose.

The head is steady; face—imperturbable; eyes—aware; neck—secure; torso—tranquil; shoulders—unemotional; arms—impersonal; hands—intelligent; fingers—knowing; waist—accommodating; pelvis—cooperative; spine—assured; legs—significant; feet—responsive; elbows and knees—willing; wrists and ankles—acquiescent.

Physiologically, the total body with its distinctive attributes, is dual in nature.

The body is "divided" into two sections. The upper part—torso and head—is yin, and the lower—pelvis and legs—yang. The waistline is the area of separation. Each part acts with contrasting intensities to balance the forces of power and lightness, of energy and release. The lower section carries the body's weight and firmly holds all movement and changes with strength in gravitational balance. The upper section, supported as it is by the power of pelvis and legs, is light, passive and quiet as if it were weightless. The torso is always free of intense tension, protecting heart and lungs from undue muscular pressure. The head retains its lightness and steadiness throughout the many changes of form and dynamics of the rest of the body. It remains 'light-headed,' no burden to neck or shoulders, never succumbing to the force of gravity. With head upright and shoulders relaxed, the spine can retain a correctly balanced form, even as it is moved and stretched by continual pelvis action.

To keep the dual aspects of the body functioning and feeling as one, the muscular energy must be distributed correctly, i.e., intrinsically, at all times. The dynamic demands for using 'force' differ for various parts of the body, depending on muscle-joint relationships as well as on structural patterns, combinations of forms and angle of space direction.

The natural (intrinsic) power which keeps the body stable in terms of gravity lies in the pelvic region, supported by the legs. The torso with head, shoulders and arms need never use any force even remotely resembling the intensity which must be exerted by the legs. The ranges of muscular-dynamic changes also differ enormously, the upper region always remaining proportionately light, with the help of the power of the lower region.

Within each region there are varieties and degrees of light and strong dynamic interplay which are in no way paralleled in the other. An obvious example is that the intense power needed to maintain a standing position on one leg alone need not be duplicated when lifting an arm in the air. This exemplifies the intrinsic use of energy. One would not remain upright for very long were the legs to try to use as little energy as is required by the arms to function. When too much airiness (lightness) outweighs the force needed for stability. then one is vulnerable. When the strong force outweighs and eliminates the light unnecessarily, then one is brutal.

Structure regulates the body's dualities by balancing the yin-yang elements with their form, direction, mass-line, tempo variations, and space-designed geometrical patterns. When all elements are counter-poised in proper proportion and are therefore cooperating in space and time, we can be assured that the physical *certainty* will produce emotional equilibrium and mental ease.

The physical and mental aspects are developed and cultivated as one at the same time. Physical culture in t'ai-chi ch'üan implies mental culture, since mental activity is awareness of the process of execution. Little, except for the instinctive and mechanical, "happens" to the body unless the mind-will is there and alert to move it. Cooperatively, we have mental agility and physical energy, mental energy and physical agility— interchangeably. The body and mind are in partnership. This duality— the complementary opposites—can be resolved. For its fundamental safety, the body must willingly unite itself with the mind's way. In a flash they can be 'as one', because body exercises mind and mind the body.

Mind-body duality is of greater importance than the instinctive duality of the yin-yang physical body. The centered mind directs the harmony of the dual-self by calling attention to what is happening, and to what is to come. The mind acting with the body makes the body act with itself. The mind becomes one with the action and the body acts as one with the mind. These dualities are the functioning features of the one totality, many 'ones' forming a single one. . . "The Supreme Ultimate".

Mind cannot exist without a body, but body can "live" or exist with *no* mind but on a low level of existence as when a body in a coma carries on with "no" mind activity. ("It is the mind that makes the body rich."—Shakespeare.) When the body is stirred by and seems to be one with mind, then action attains a conscious ease which becomes ingrained, as if it were second nature. Nevertheless, the mind must be the "over-see-er" since the physical body, when left to itself, will "copy itself"—that is, repeat what it had already done despite the changing situation which only the mind can be capable of knowing. If the body is left to itself, certain habits become automatic, eventually useless and destructive. Consciously made habits, on the contrary, protect the system; when they cease to be useful, they can be changed or washed out by mind's insistence.

The t'ai-chi ch'üan player, aware and completely centered on what is being done, gives the impression of "careless" ease. The sum of all the opposites—yin and yang dynamics, the dual nature of body physiology, mind-body/internal/external experience—produces an appearance of weightlessness, a result of mind-body discipline and impeccable balance. The observer sees the "by-product" of such discipline. The player experiences and is changed by the complete action, to become and remain calm. Impressed by its outer appearance, the observer reacts to the "aesthetics" of t'ai-chi ch'üan, and feels an agreeable calm. The *real* nature of the exercise is the inner essence, feeling and awareness on all levels, which emanates from functioning with centered mind, disciplined body and correct form.

No one has analyzed the Yin-Yang duality of observer and "doer" more succinctly than *Wu Chien Ch'üan* and *Ma Yüeh-Liang* in their book entitled *T'ai-Chi Ch'üan* (Shanghai 1935.) I quote (in a shortened version) their comparison of the internal aspects and external appearances of t'ai-chi ch'üan:

1.   seems airy—but has substance and is weighted; action "is like refined steel"
2.   seems thoughtless—but is attentive and concentrated; "spirit is like a cat waiting to catch a mouse"
3.   seems soft and easy—but it is controlled "like pulling silk out of a cocoon"
4.   seems as if there were no dynamics—but inner variations of dynamics are like the "movement flow of a river"
5.   the outside looks reposeful and effortless—inside is firm and stable
6.   there is a reserve of energy like a "bow about to be snapped"

The constancy of the mind and the consistency of the body manipulation are the two great simultaneous "ones." This connected body-self and mindful-self span and integrate the emotional and the intellectual selves.

Health and philosophy are one in t'ai-chi ch'üan. It is a wise mind that knows its own body; it is a wise body that knows its own mind. And together they make a most satisfactory state to be in and to live with.

## II. Way of the Mind: Tranquil Power

Mind, the constant principle in the activity of t'ai-chi ch'üan, is concerned with the conduct of the body both for the *body's* sake, and for its own superior development. Not only is t'ai-chi ch'üan a 'from the mind' exercise but it is a 'with and for the mind' technique. In acting 'with' the mind, a state of awareness brings both attention to and appreciation of what is experienced continually. 'For' the mind indicates that it is possible to improve one's faculties and to attain a high level of consciousness and perception. The Method becomes more refined, subtle, profound and practical as mind directs the body to function with increasing perfection, physically and mentally.

Mind is always multiply engaged: it observes and reacts; responds and directs; evaluates and leads; it initiates and experiences. At the same time, it serves itself in the process, augmenting its own potential powers—never remaining at the same level of ability. This is the mind of the Meaning.

Although mind seems to move from place to place as if it were not doing anything, it functions with clearly directed energy. Ever-present attention is the prevailing element which prevents the body from acting mechanically and automatically. Even in the most ordinary of everyday movements, as in walking, the mind must be present, alert for any contingency—evaluating the situation and redirecting action when necessary. Were mind not present, however faintly, at all times—unforeseen occurrences could not be taken care of successfully. When mind is trained to be alive to outer circumstances in relation to the self, the measure of timed reaction between mind and body is infinitessimal.

At every step of the way of this exceedingly complex structure, the mind prepares the continuous way by adhering to the immediate, the *now* of the situation. Mind, being one and with the moment, senses the future with the aid of memory—coordinating sensations, distinguishing and combining them. When mind falters and misses the present moment, it misses the most significant space-time connection flowing into the "future".

Mind does not function on a one-track road, which would limit 'vision' and understanding of the possibility of mind's own further development. Mind sees, knows, and manipulates a multitude of facts at once. Just as the eyes when focused on a centered dot can see everything within the periphery of its vision, so the mind perceives not one 'item' but the entire range of the specifically coordinated ingredients of action and thought. Mind functions with the related and coherent activities of the instant—from the nuance of dynamics to the interlinear movements, all at the instant of the coordination of the relevant component parts. Mind can comprehend the quality of the 'stillness' and progression of action and the power of its own presence.

The unique, composite nature of the composition (described in the way of structure, page 164) channels the mind and compels it to remain awake and ready to act with speed. It is the nature of the structured exercise not to permit mind to abandon the body—to sacrifice it for its own fantasies.

Attention is centered on the act itself as mind organizes and coordinates the processes, which are never elementary. In so doing the mind trains itself to stick to and perceive the most minute of changes. Through its efforts the body is eased into the most delicate of combinations which are necessary physiologically for impeccable balance. As the mind directs, the body responds to the everchanging form-patterns. It evaluates the basic tempo and the slowed-up tempi simultaneously. It creates the continuity of the sustained flow of movement. It appreciates the interweaving dynamic qualities of the individual units and knows the harmonious correctness of the activity—remaining objective and unperturbed by the constant interchange of greater or lesser complexities. If by any chance it has abstracted itself from the physical action, it is soon brought back to the 'subject' by the body's incorrect motion, which would inevitably be made without mind's help. Body aids the mind, even inadvertently.

With the body, mind shares the depths of the coordinated process. The way of the mind can comprehend all and share with the body a unity of experience. Mind is everywhere, like the air.

However, mind must be "willing", which is to say that a person must have the will 'power' to persevere—to help the mind rid itself of irrelevant thoughts. From concentrating and being-with the act of moving in this most orderly of compositions arises an agreeable sense of physical ease and mental quiet.

As mind processes the interrelationship of form, space, time and dynamics, the motion of mind also moves into the 'realm' of the heart and its emotions. Mind can instantly detect a change of 'heart', for better or worse. When mind is in a dilemma, the heart is uneasy; when thoughts are settled, the heart is soothed.

Then it is no paradox to say that the heart of the matter of t'ai-chi ch'üan is the mind, since it is the way of mind that leads the heart to equanimity and helps the heart to be mindful of itself. Perhaps it can also be said that the mind of the matter is in the heart, since both interact mentally and emotionally.

The Chinese do not separate heart and mind by individual words: their one word *hsin* for heart and mind implies that each has an effect on the other, positively or negatively, and does not act separately. For the Chinese, "to lose the soul of the mind" is to be greatly frightened. We in the West say "frightened out of our wits." In both metaphors, the mind is obliterated by emotion.

The concept of heart-mind 'as one,' may or may not imply that heart and mind are equals on all occasions. In the philosophy of t'ai-chi ch'üan: the greater power for man's development lies in the consciousness of the mind which produces heart calmness; the heart must listen to the mind; it is possible to become exceedingly sensitive to the most fleeting of emotional reactions; the mind, in "minding all", protects the body from destroying itself emotionally and falling into a rut of unproductive habits.

The way mind relates to the harmonious structure puts body on an even keel of physical security and emotional stability by conserving energy and soothing the nervous system. Brought to life are the many facets of the Meaning—patience, perseverance, endurance, and equilibrium of thought and action. Permanently present, mind progresses to greater depths of astuteness, with insight as to man's potentiality, eventually to comprehend the "Ultimate Meaning."

The individual aspects of action and mind synthesize into a 'unity of oneness', just as the colors of the rainbow fuse into a unity—the *whiteness* of light. At the final moment of the exercise, mind and body seem to 'disappear' and become something 'other', created by their intrinsic, harmonious cooperation. The quality of the sensation is one of lightness, and contained vitality.

The t'ai-chi ch'üan way of mind's tranquil power develops the patience of a scientist and creates the patience of a saint.

Structure is all and everything. It is the Mind of the Body and The Minding Body. It is the concrete physiological configurations and abstractions of time and space. It is a harmony of aesthetics and mathematics, mental discipline and feeling. It is moving-form and changing-stillness. It is process (Becoming) and purpose (Being) simultaneously. It is substance and spirit. Structure is the ch'üan of the T'ai-chi and the T'ai-chi way of the ch'üan. Never deviating from the organic laws of nature, t'ai-chi ch'üan is a triumph of ingenuity and insight as to the way man can develop himself fully.

The appearance of the structured action is as flowingly still as a smooth horizon which unites and yet outlines the quiet of the sky and the stirring of the sea. The even and steady curvilinear way of t'ai-chi ch'üan movement (like a horizon) defines with great clarity the intricately detailed Forms while blending with the action to make a unified whole.

The leading interacting aspects of this structured whole are (1) its physical harmony: how the bodily organization remains in and achieves equilibrium in the continual act of changing positions, and (2) its structural harmony: the formal arrangements of the action-structure which relate basically to the superior development of complete mental, emotional and physical health.

The structure is a balanced synthesis of Body-Space-Time: of all the organic changes, of the designed constructions and of the gravitational interacting dynamics of energy and formed-motion. The perfection of the precisely composed composition of t'ai-chi ch'üan makes Meaning come to life, simultaneous with the action.

The total body, in no matter what formal movement, is always in correct alignment and dynamic balance, each part functioning with the others intrinsically. Every position is spaced and timed so as to be concretely perceived and felt as a unit. The connections from one place to another, bodily or spatially, are discerned and experienced as being regulated with structured logic and physical consistency, each position giving way to another with comfortable ease.

No gesture is arbitrary, accidental or wilfully improvised. Every movement is appreciated as coming at the right time, for the right reason. Everything in t'ai-chi ch'üan, the slightest turn of the hand or angle of the head, has been designed and composed with mathematical exactness, philosophical sensitivity, and physical validity—thus relating each and every movement harmoniously to the total conception.

Just as a wall structure would be weakened by the removal of a brick, so the t'ai-chi ch'üan movements, which are always structural, cannot be altered, tampered with, or omitted without destroying the *integrity* and power of the exercise and its essential Meaning.

The structure is composed of 108 significant Forms and their connecting Transitions. These Forms "contain" great ideological power, and yet in the unending continuity of motion they appear with "modesty", and with no more apparent emphasis than do the innumerable patterned transitions. In the *flow* of action, all are equally considered, but in the *structure* of the action, the Forms each have a profound individuality (to be discussed later). However, the motion keeps all in a steady pace to the last moment of the final stillness, no matter how much the internal dynamics and external patterns vary .

Each Form symbolizes a state of being or becoming and therefore represents a concept, an aim—in the goals of the Meaning—as for instance patience, centered attention, consciousness, wisdom. Each Form is "disguised" by a metaphorical name, such as "Grasping the Bird's Tail", "Hand Strums the Lute", "The Golden Needle at the Bottom of the Deep Sea"—symbolic and allegorical names.

It is necessary to state here that only when one has "lived" with the exercise and has achieved a state of proficiency are the real meanings of the Forms revealed. When one has reached a state of awareness and can be truly centered, and possesses patience, the Meanings will be more than intellectual words, which they are at the beginning of study. When one is ready and prepared, the Meaning has intrinsic life and essence.

In the Wu Style, the 25 to 30 minute t'ai-chi ch'üan structure has six series or divisions. At each level a more advanced stage in the evolutionary process of self-development is revealed, both structurally and meaningfully. These series, continuing without visible halts, are perceived from the point of view of physical progress, emotional stability and mental agility. And the unity in this multiple process is always maintained, evident and experienced.

The quality which distinguishes bodily organization is perpetual physiological balance, as it relates to form, movement, patterns and design. All muscles and joints in the structural changes of head, torso, pelvis and legs remain in perfect alignment, whatever the shape of Transitions, the frame of the Forms, direction of movement, and the dynamics of energy.

Perfect balance through the proper distribution of the forces and proportions of the body—in space and time—awakens a feeling of complete lightness and stability, at *all* times.

All positions, spaced and timed, are perceived and felt tangibly. The movement connections from place to place, subtle or obvious, are discerned as being regulated with utmost body-form logic, with almost imperceptible smoothness—each part of the body giving way to another position, less or more intricately composed, with inevitable ease. The always changing patterns and movements stimulate and rest different parts of the body in turn, each being definite as to placement and dynamics. With mind directing, the exact space-form positions improve body sensitivity, stamina, coordination and perceptiveness of the harmony of the self.

An aspect of the way of structure is the harmonious integration of all its elements—no matter how combined. The elements that distinguish the *formal arrangements* are position, pattern, space, direction, movement, dynamics of energy (yin-yang), dynamics of proportion of form and tempo. These factors integrate and interact in various ways, and are simultaneously present at each and every moment. All are responsible for the balance of the whole, no one factor being isolated. Their impeccable interrelationship controls the harmony and so *is* the harmony of structure.

Though each element may combine with others in dozens of ways, the following show how some may interact with and "mutually help" others.

1. Changing positions combine with dynamics of movement
2. Dynamics of movement depend on form
3. Form combines with space
4. Space-form depends on tempo
5. Tempo depends on coordination
6. Coordination influences attention
7. Attention controls body-action
8. Body-action determines energy-dynamics (yin-yang)
9. Yin-yang depends on gravity and changing positions

Different relationships of the elements can be accepted as being equally valid: that coordination affects position and position direction; that direction determines space and space regulates form, etc. Cause and effect can be balanced in many ways since t'ai-chi ch'üan is an integrated and perpetually changing harmony of action, physiology, and structure.

Ordered diversity can be shown to exist in any Form-Transition structure. The following analysis of the Flying Oblique Form illustrates the harmony of its balanced proportions in terms of its diversity. (Figure 222)

222

Legs are placed in a northeast-southwest diagonal, setting the torso to the northwest; the parallel feet point to northwest. The space between the feet is wide, resulting from the deep kneebend of the preceding position. Torso bends forward slightly; the pelvis is contracted. (Never is the bending torso placed parallel to the ground.) The left knee is bent holding 70% of the weight and the right leg is straight. Torso is pulled over to the left side which is strong (yang); this left side is balanced by the yin of the outstretched left arm held at shoulder height, with palm upturned (yin). The right side of the straight right leg is yin; parallel to it is the straight right arm; palm facing down, wrist flexed (yang), is slightly in front of right knee. The right fingers point to northeast; left fingers point west. The head, held slightly downward, is turned to northeast; eyes look at back of right hand.

Space-form-dynamics-position-direction are so balanced that the "sum" of the Form produces a sensation of lightness; this is also true of every "passing" transition. Structurally, the lightness is *in* the unity — the balance of all elements as they move or rest — which dominates totally. The intrinsic process unfailingly evokes calmness, patience, serenity and awareness. The Meaning, when experienced, transforms the organic material into "spirit".

The following chapter contains a detailed analysis of the intrinsic, organic and objective features of the structure, the creative synthesis of which constitutes the Exercise-Art of t'ai-chi ch'üan.

## CHAPTER 8

*1. The Frame of Space-Composition*

The exercise moves within a clearly defined ground space, the dimensions of which have been created by the structure itself—the combination of moving form-patterns and physiological balance. See the Foot Chart at the back of this book.

The over-all area has been proportioned to be a seven by fourteen foot rectangle—the foot not being scaled by the 12 inches of the ruler but by the *personal* foot length of the player. The actual size of the rectangle varies also according to the length of the individual's stepping-space; however it will always be in correct proportion for each person since the 'seven by fourteen' relationship never varies structurally.

The paths the foot patterns traverse, changing frequently, move in the eight directions of the compass: north (*facing front*), (south) to the rear, (east) to the right and west (to the left) and the diagonals, northeast and northwest, southeast and southwest. The floor space can be visualized as being 98 (7 by 14) foot squares. The relationship of form to space is mathematically exact.

The axis line of this area goes from east to west and is placed two squares from the rear south boundary. Note that the full space is divided into a 2 by 5 proportion, the front part being five squares long, north to south (front to back). Awareness of this axis line is important; it is the centering reference point for all that occurs in passing from one place to another; also, the exercise begins and ends in the same square of this axis-line. (page 227). This fact is significant in terms of having the physical ability to maintain correct proportion of body and leg positions, as well as philosophically, in perceiving that the 'ending' is a 'new' beginning. When this "end" position is achieved, it proves that the foot movement manipulation has been relatively perfect in respect to floor plan, design and space-direction.

The intrinsic world of the self is directed to function with the outside world of geographical space—the 'plan' of the active body configurations reacting to the demands of space. The various combinations of the composition are directed to function with the 'world' of the body : the 'plan' of the Forms is based on the nature of the physiological way. Since t'ai-chi ch'üan is a unity of what takes place in the body system and its movements, the accuracy of spaced floor placements depends not on legs and feet alone but also on the action of all body formations since the relationship of torso, pelvis, and arms also determine how controlled, accurate, and balanced the legs can be in their designed positions.

All motion is harmoniously constructed to take place in stipulated areas. Even the most minute turn of the toe is regulated by the position of the body to balance with the form of the space. Awareness of how movement is made and balance achieved inevitably leads to the correct, impeccable final position—that of ending at the original 'footprint' space-stance.

## 2. The Value of Tempo Variation

It has already been noted (page 34) that an unwavering basic tempo prevails throughout t'ai-chi ch'üan: some part of the body actively continues the tempo even if only by a simple hand movement or turn of the head. Within the basic tempo other tempi vary in degrees of slowness or speed. Moving more slowly than basic time is intrinsically controlled; moving faster is being extrinsic since tensed force is necessary to form the quickened positions.

### (1) Slowed-Up Tempi

Slowed-up tempi are not always in the *same* time-span. Since the structural configurations are complex, various parts of the body are made to move in different tempi in order to arrive at the designated coordinated position simultaneously.

Space and time are inextricably related as point 26 in Chapter 2 shows. The simple exercise indicates that in rendering a set form the larger spaced action always continues in basic tempo, while movements covering smaller areas are slowed up in proportion to the size of the space traversed.

It is my belief that it is the nuances and the subtle variations of the slowed-up tempi within the ever-changing shapes that produce a tranquil feeling and an atmosphere of "perpetual" motion. Repetitive timing throughout would easily result in both mechanically made movement and in a weakening of mind attention. The many changes in the slowed-up tempo processes—sometimes requiring legs to slow up, other times the arms or torso—demand constant and intent attention for impeccable coordination. This contributes to the development of patience and to tranquility as well.

### (2) Speeded-up Action

There are *nine* places where the tempo changes from the regulated slow basic time to speeded-up flashes of action. These are considered extrinsic since a gathering of extra force in the body is necessary to make the quickened gestures. The more speedily done, the greater the prowess to move from the basic slow tempo. The changes demand quick thinking and challenges physical and mental alertness. Resumption of the slow tempo is also part of the discipline of being able to command the body to follow any change of thought-command.

The speeded-up patterns are all different except for one which is a repeat, so that mind's attention is constantly active. For instance, in Series III, there are three different flashes of speed: in Form 40 one quick toe turn moves the body 90° (page 81); in Form 42 the total body moves with arms and legs in action; and in Form 52 the body rotates in a 180° turn (from north to south). The ninth quick movement (Form 106) is of special interest since the torso and legs continue to move slowly while the arms make a single rapid movement (see page 145). This Form epitomizes the necessity of developing superior ability to move with force and speed without disturbing the calm of the slow-tempo of the moving body. To do so is to accomplish a simultaneous balance of tensed extrinsic speed in one part of the body and soft intrinsic slowness in the rest of one body. In the evolutionary development of the self such coordinated action is a symbol for having the power to deal with and to conquer adverse conditions with equanimity.

The quick movements do not affect the breathing tempo when there is mental preparedness for the physical activity.

The rapid movements will never become automatic. They will always demand 'pulled together' energy, and 'yang' mental attention. Recognition of these 'isolated' details is a source of gratification and contributes to the appreciation of what is always to be experienced—that the diversity of events in t'ai-chi ch'üan—movement, form, space and tempo—become a "unit" of harmonious action.


### 3. The Organic Nature of Shapes and Shades of Movement

Intrinsic to the way of movement is its style—that of the ever-flowing action, even and light, balanced and slow, moving in heart-beat tempo. Although these characteristics can be loosely present in any kind of physical activity, in t'ai-chi ch'üan they are interwoven into the fabric and construction of the structure, and contribute to the meaningful accomplishment of calmness and equilibrium.

Shape: The dominating factor in the composition of the whole is that of the curving elements. All possible variations of curvilinear movement are present in the shapes (forms) and the shades (dynamics) of the action— arc, oval, wave, parabola, spiral, circle, hook and hair-pin turn.

The fundamental shape, *and* the most important, is the combination of the circle and the wave, synchronized to reflect the T'ai-chi symbol.

223

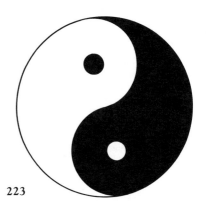

The circle-waves of action are formed in such a way as *never* to be a literal rendition of reality, which would be to make a *complete* circle form and a full wave line. They are rendered as symbolic segments—implying circle and wave stylistically—i.e. a quarter of a circle, made with one arm, embracing or enclosing an undulating form resembling a wave, made by the other.

Circle-wave forms can be made horizontally or vertically and can be small as passing movements or large as a Form. They are always centered at middle thorax (chest) level, and held at least 9 inches away from it. Used both as Transition and Form they are always balanced by the proper placements of the leg positions.

Form 1, named the T'ai-Chi (see page 41), is a perfect example of the vertical circle-wave combination. The circle is indicated by the raised left arm with palm facing the forehead; the right hand is placed at heart level, the palm facing outward, with the angle of the right elbow and the bent wrist forming a wavelike curve. Ninety-five percent of the body's weight is on the bent right leg; the left is outstretched resting lightly on the heel. The shades of the dynamics and the shape of the Form are exactly balanced in space-mass aspects.

When joined with a 'wave' the circle surrounding it is conceived to be 'completeness', limiting the space in which the wave activity can move. Symbolically the circle is 'stillness', like that of a mountain, and the wave is activity, like that of a flowing river. They make a unity of opposites, physiologically (materially) and philosophically (spiritually). T'ai-chi is "an urge to wholeness in the flight of changing phenomena" (Dyson). T'ai-chi is "mind, the Supreme Ultimate" (Ma Yüeh-Liang).

The organic nature of body movement is curve—one cannot but move in curves: in turning a circle is made; lifting an arm describes an arc; shifting toes while pivoting on heel makes an arc as does any movement of the head. Subtleties of structure, like manipulation of a hand, have to be mind attended. Unwavering attention, concentration on the act of moving, and living with the ever-varying space-shapes awakens an interesting sensation of 'magnetism'. The more minute the movement, the greater is circulation to sensitive parts of the body, and with it the further progress of a sensitive mind.

In addition to the curvilinear process there is the 'straight-line' shape. Generally singly made in any direction—vertical, horizontal, and oblique— they are usually joined to moving arc-shapes and, like the wave-line patterns, take place within the area of the curve spaces. Depending on the space to be covered in order simultaneously to end a form, each separately may be in basic or slowed-up time. Straight line action, being more difficult to perceive than the dominating curvilinear process, demands more concentrated attention, thereby furthering the power of the mind.

The straight and the curved lines move in special ways in relation to space and contain subtle variations of dynamics within the formed gesture. The dynamic variations come from the pattern and designs, the directions of movements which move away and toward the body, up and down, in and out, forward or backward—going with or against gravity. All are dynamically different: the light, the strong and the many shades of yin and yang in between. An example of a straight-spaced gesture will illustrate the relationship of form and direction. Bend the left elbow and place it at the side of the body; bend arm so that wrist is close to shoulder; bend wrist, palm down, pointing fingers forward. Move arm parallel to floor so that finger tips lead the action, full length at shoulder height. In so doing the wrist is being straightened, making the entire arm feel light in contrast to the original position, which was strong. This illustrates moving in a *straight line*, with the changing form determining the strong and light dynamics.

Energy changes also depend on and include positions in relation to the pull of gravity, positions in large or small units staying at one level or departing from it. Any angle of direction with pattern will shade the dynamic use of energy in such a balanced and harmonious way that the resultant Form will feel 'light', as well as the transitory movements.

The intrinsic shapes and shades of changing movements permit the body to endure the activity without effort for longer and longer consecutive periods of time. Endurance and stamina, physical and mental, easily develop with the organic nature of balanced, flowing changes.

The entire body, from head to toe—every joint, every muscle, with mind and feeling, is involved in performing and responding to the movements. A significant 'part' of the body not yet emphasized is the eyes. Just as the muscles of the body are manipulated with strength and lightness, through the action of form and space, so do the muscles of the eyes behave, in a similar intrinsic manner.

In looking at a distant object or a close one, the eye muscles adjust naturally to the space changes—more tensely when the object is close and lightly when it is distant. During most of the exercise eyes are 'held' naturally and neutrally—looking at some point about 15 feet away from the positioned feet. Focussing in this way the eyelids are partially lowered without any tenseness as the eyes look out on a downward slanted path. This is the eye position when not specifically directed to look at the palm, fingertips, or back of hand—which may be at different times close to or outstretched a full arm length from the body.

In Cloud Arms Form (Form 32), the designs call for the eyes to look at the variously positioned hand placements. Thus eye muscles are lightly or strongly activated. For instance, one hand is placed eye high about 12 inches in front of the eyes, which are "forced" at this distance to open wide, thus tensely activating the muscles. (Figure 224) At another point, the hand is lowered, releasing the eye tension. The Form patterns are repeated with the eye movements being alternately adjusted to have tension and release. At the end of this Form the eyes are directed to look far away into space, by which action eye muscles are completely rested. The dynamic

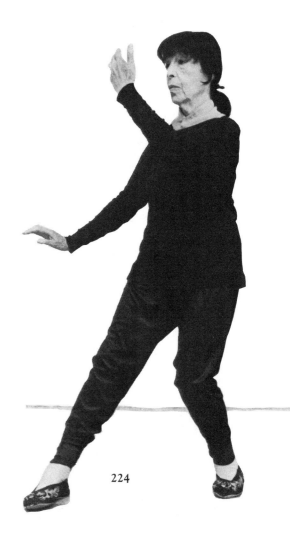

224

shades of eye movement function with the Form as consistently and naturally as does any other part of the body. The shapes of Form determine the shades of the dynamics.

The eyes are at 'ease', even when specially activated. They do not peer, gaze or strain to "see," but behave as the ears do—which just 'hear'; the eyes must just "see". Needless to say, the eyes have a most difficult task, since they reflect every and any emotion—fear, anger, anxiety, suspicion, etc.—which not only put the eye muscles into extrinsically tensed action but which also affect the facial ones. Since in t'ai-chi ch'üan negative emotions are eventually erased by the 'impersonal' objective action, the eyes can remain calm and function intrinsically, *all the time.*

The Chinese call the eyes "the cottage of the spirit" since they reveal personality. With the elimination of negative emotions, a goal in this non-subjective exercise, the spirit revealed will be that of equanimity.

## 4. The Integrity of Shapes and Shades of Form and Transition

The body experiences and the mind senses that each of the 108 Forms is a culmination of a set of interweaving themes termed "Transition". The mind perceives the moment of unity as if time had ceased to be. The body holding the Form feels the integrated synthesis of dynamics, space, direction and design. These diverse elements can be said to have been neutralized into a stilled moment. Just as two complementary colors—as red and green—when mixed in proper proportions become a different color (gray-neutral), so the progressive blending of the complementary elements of a specific transition leads to and creates Form, a new dimension in the evolving stages of Meaning.

Because, for a fraction of an instant, a Form appears to be unmoving, it produces a feeling of having arrived at a journey's end. The body, nevertheless, is not static or grounded, since the body-mind system is intrinsically alert and always latently prepared to move into action.

Each Form instigates the action of a Transition-theme which in turn leads to another Form. These alternating sequences continue throughout the entire structure, each achieving its balance in opposite ways. Whereas in the Transition all elements are in constant motion, transforming space with tempo, dynamics with physiological manipulations, in Form all such distinctions evaporate and a unique unit of completion is created.

Transition is considered to be yang; Form is yin. Transition is the harmony of action—the 'Means'; Form is the harmony of stillness—the 'Ends'. In the overall picture of the Grand Structure, the Transition activity beginning the exercise is yang; the Form which concludes the exercise, stillness and quiescence, is yin.

The names of each of the 108 Forms are symbolic and allegorically profound, never literally representational. Each is a meaningfully directed indication of what is to be finally awakened and understood philosophically in terms of the goals, and what is to be achieved in respect to the body-mind's progress in the development of physical and emotional stability.

It is said that each Form is a 'station', a state of being, on the road to higher consciousness. Each Form symbolizes and highlights one of the many Meanings (see page 154). It is not the Form itself but the entire exercise as a continuum which gradually gives insight into various stages of heart-mind equilibrium. Comprehension of oneself grows throughout the exercise as a whole, as each Transition-process moves into a Form. Only when one has already acquired a modicum of calmness, patience and concentration do the Forms become individually and conceptually significant. Therefore, it is customary *not* to reveal the true Meanings of the symbolically named Forms until such time as the player has acquired, without thinking about it, certain insights into the essential values, through deeply-felt experience. It is inevitable that this *will* happen without any self-conscious intellectualization during the activity.

As has been noted above, all Forms are yin and Transitions, yang. Within this dominating category of the yin-yang family, there are further differences to be experienced and recognized which also have a dual relationship—which might be called 'lesser' yins and yangs.

Within the 108 Form (yin) group there are two subdivisions called *Hsü* (meaning void) and *Shih* (solid-full). These are descriptive terms and when used in the whole exercise, they refer to the dynamics of weightedness and lightness; the more and the less active strengths. All positions partake of this duality, which is the balance of different energies.

When Forms are designated as *Hsü* or *Shih*, the concepts are abstract symbols of quality—not physical. *Hsü* Forms are those which have abstract meanings of wisdom, consciousness, equanimity. *Shih* Forms are those which imply concrete firmness, power, steadfastness. With a few exceptions, these Forms appear in alternating sequences throughout.

The names of T'ai-chi and the Ch'üan similarly embrace both the abstract and concrete: Ch'üan being solid (as matter) and T'ai-chi being void (as spirit). Together they constitute the mental-physical, the abstract-concrete, the intangible-tangible harmony.

Although I believe that awareness of and insight into Meanings are experienced by *living* (with) the exercise, I nevertheless do not hesitate to offer a few illustrations of void and solid qualities—even if by so doing, some of the inner Meanings will be partially revealed. This is inevitable, since it is Meaning, not the symbolic name, which reflects its void or solid nature. These aspects, too, are interwoven in the chain of the alternating yin-yang process along with the changing dynamics of energy and structure, space, and direction.

The process of action beginning the exercise flows from simple symmetry to a complex harmony of dynamics, patterns, space and direction, giving 'birth' to Form T'ai-Chi—the essence of harmonious relationships. This Form symbolizes the "completion of the world" from which solid fact other and higher centers of man can develop. A complex Transition then follows, which culminates in *Hsü* (void) Form—Grasping the Bird's Tail.

The Single Whip Form is solid, aiming as it does for strength, firmness and stamina. Transitions preceding it being relatively simple. All Forms and Transitions are experienced without necessarily noting the alternating process of conceptual variations. All action at every moment is harmoniously in balance, even though with knowledge the entire exercise is experienced as being yin and yang, the void and the solid shades and shapes in alternation.

Transitions are like grammatically variegated sentences—structures which open the way to abstract concepts and concrete facts of action. Ever changing, the 108 Transitions are the life-giving material of t'ai-chi ch'üan, containing through rich diversity the means to achieve body health, mind awareness, containment and consciousness.

Transitions differ in degrees of complexity and length and vary in the technique of how curve, space, time and line of direction relate to each other. Short or long, the complex Transitions increase the need to concentrate, to develop the power to maintain physical balance and to sensitize perception of detailed connections. The simple Transitions ease up and reduce mind and body effort. The alternating rhythm of 'more or less work' physically and mentally, carries out the basic tenets so that at no point throughout this exercise is any part of the body overstrained, overworked and exhausted.

Because the structural relationships are mathematically and technically integrated—down to the very second—all in accordance with the physiological laws of nature as well as the philosophical principles of cause and effect, no Forms or Transitions may be omitted, altered or rearranged *if* the ultimate Meaning is to come to life and be finally realized.

Forms and Transitions exist together side by side in continuity, and their 'differences' are always harmoniously felt. The balance of their structural unity in completion is exemplified by the fact that the ending Form (void) is exactly the same in body position as the beginning (Transition) position, which is the 'potential' for the first Form *T'ai-Chi* (solid). The ending Form stands in the same "foot-prints" as the beginning. These positions, though similar externally, are immensely different in spirit and quality.

When starting the exercise, one is seemingly innocent as to what develops. This is true every time one begins the exercise. The beginning stance is a preparation for action; the final Form is rich with the experience of mind-body unity and has the feeling of fulfillment, in contrast to the beginning action, which is one of anticipation.

The ending contains as well the 'presence' of a *new* beginning on a higher level of consciousness. One can *never*, although one is in the correct structured footsteps, begin the exercise again immediately. The spirit of the ending and beginning are worlds apart. The shapes and shades of Form and Transition have passed through involved and varied complexities to arrive at a higher stage—that of 'oneness'—where Form has become Content-Meaning.

Not only for reasons relating to physical-mental ease, memory and awareness are themes repeated; also vitally important is the concept that the differences in time and place in which repeats arise are factors in arousing a profound change in "content". Thus for instance a Hand Strums the Lute Form which is made to the west and a similar one made to the east (compare Forms 9 and 61) contain subtle changes in feeling.

Many of the 108 Forms appear time and time again in various areas of the floor space: The Single Whip—nine times; Grasping the Bird's Tail Form— seven times; High Pat the Horse Form—five times—to mention but a few. What is especially pertinent is that each and every repetition has its own distinct significance. Not *one* repetition can be eliminated without destroying the sense and the integrity of the whole structure. Were this not so, each Form would merely be a matter of physical-body-design, irrespective of its being repeated and of the necessity for its exact placement— the omission of which would affect the entire composition, mathematically as well as spiritually.

Being more than a physical unit, Form progresses and grows in 'content' each time it is repeated. Such organic development is attributed to: (l) where it appears in the frame of the floor-space areas; (2) in which direction it appears in the eightsided 'landscape'; (3) in which of the six series it is formed again; (4) the nature of the interacting sequences and what issues from it; (5) the awareness of the quality of stamina and ease, awakened in the evolutionary cycle of the whole.

Although the Single Whip Form is directed to the same north-west angle seven times out of nine, it never appears in the same space. This Form follows the Grasping the Bird's Tail seven times, and Cloud Arms twice. It cannot be taken for granted, however, since what leads from it is subtly, minutely different—the first six times being new connections, the remaining three being repeats. Decidedly the attention must be alert to space and place. If mind strays, the body out of unthinking habit reverts to an earlier and already performed pattern-sequence.

Although what *follows* Grasping the Bird's Tail Form is always the same— the Single Whip Form— what leads *into* it is *always* different and requires special attention each time. The transitions leading into it vary in tempi directing arm-leg relationships and weight-coordinated balances. However, taking less thought, the ending of this Form is the same repeated pattern which always leads to the Single Whip. For the 'Bird' Form, then, what leads *into* it is of great mental concern, whereas with the Single Whip, in contrast, what leads *from* it demands more concentration. These complex and simple sequences illustrate the way mind application varies in degree of intensity—light-Yin and deep-Yang efforts— whether 'lessened or intensified'. The mind 'changes' according to the action's diverse problems.

Structural differentiations contribute to the comprehension both of how the physical body need never expend its energy and of how the mind responds to the process of perpetual change without tiring. Psychologically Cloud Arms Form is so easy-going (and seductive) that the mind takes-off, letting the body carry on mechanically by itself. Like a faint and transparent cloud, this Form can evaporate, leaving no trace of its presence in the memory. When this occurs, thoughts and emotions (generally unpleasant) float up from the unconscious and momentarily disconcert one. They disappear when the mind comes back, spurred on by a different sequence. If a "thought" is remembered at the conclusion of the exercise, it can be dealt with intellectually, with the calmness and patience accumulated during the progress of the consecutive and conscious action.

When one arrives at this Cloud Arms Form the *second* time round some ten minutes later, the practitioner always "wakes up" to its existence — since a greater ability to concentrate has been developing with the variety of the ever new action.

What often comes to mind with the repetition of this Form is a doubt as to whether it had been done the first time. This can be checked quite easily, because every position has its specific place in the space. Noting a complete change in placement would indicate that it had been omitted. The repetitions of themes, Forms and transitions are additional means to help apprise one of memory and attention lapses as well as to increase the ability to perceive and experience more subtly any instance of change.

Pitfalls are many but the more minute of changes, such as a single turn of the hand or the shifting of a foot, can jog the mind to more perceptive awareness. An example of this is the difference between the change leading from the end of the *first* Single Whip, when hands, feet and torso are redirected to make a Transition (Form 5 to 6), and the simple "solo" hand turn which leads from the Single Whip into the Transition for the Snake Creeps Down Form (from Form 78 to 79 ).

Not only do the small changing links engage the mind, but long repeated sequences require that the mind be ready for a sudden surprising small change in pattern. In the fifth series there is a repeat of a long passage of many Forms made in the second series. Such a repetition is a calming rest for mind and body; however, it tests the mind's ability to remember where one is and therefore not to lose track of the composition: to know exactly where one is in the passage of time and space.

The Right Hand Strums the Lute Form appears seven times, with only three different sequences. When the Forms that follow it are repeated many times, special effort must be made to keep the mind from wandering. Awareness of the difference of east and west contribute subtly to the "content" of the Forms.

Directing the nuances of the repetitions from lightness to intensity is of paramount importance for the development of attention, acuity and perseverance. The changes of yin-yang "ease and effort" are as vital a part of mind's growth to a higher level of consciousness as they are to the development of super-health to the body.

In all stages of the repetition of Transitions and Forms not only is the structure 'All', but necessarily the mind is "All" as well. The mind alerts the body and body the mind reciprocally, since each aspect strengthens, secures, and sharpens attention and the response to "content" in a myriad of ways.

## 6. In Perpetual Balance

Balance is the keynote of harmony. The very word conjures up the idea of a peaceful frame of mind and body-ease. These aspects are embedded in the heart of t'ai-chi ch'üan, achieved not through the word but through the balanced structure of the active process which puts body and mind into harmony. T'ai-chi ch'üan structure has been formed in such a way as to make balance absolute at every instant. 'Absolute' balance is more than physical balance alone—more than being able to perform a diversity of movements without falling over, and succumbing to gravity's pull.

In attaining physical balance, the distribution of weight is regulated, movements are coordinated, physical adjustments, requiring a certain amount of muscular strength, are made with their proper stresses.

Absolute balance implies totality of structure in all dimensions, on all fronts. The strategy of t'ai-chi ch'üan is to function in the manner of the T'ai-chi way: balancing ever-moving forms and changing dynamics in subtle grades of complexities, with time-space-volume-direction interaction in perfect accord. It can be said that gravity's power is neutralized when its own force is utilized to reassemble and rearrange relationships of forms into coordinated harmony. T'ai-chi ch'üan succeeds in making balance absolute because the power gravity exerts is always *heeded*: changes are made according to the nature of its nature. The elements of the composition are measured, combined and separated in relation to the science of how muscles and joints behave with the planned choreography which generates the Meaning.

Each exact combination produces a feeling of lightness—almost as if gravity did not exist—since the strength of physical power is balanced upward by the organization of torso, head, hands, arms, eyes, which carry the necessary yin-yang dynamics of energy and space direction. A person can be gravitationally in balance while standing on one leg (Figure 225, Form 39). In t'ai-chi ch'üan absolute balance is achieved by the way the other leg is raised, by the angle of one arm above the outstretched leg and by the direction of the other arm; how the hands are turned; where the head and eyes are directed. Every 'inch' of the total movement must be considered in terms of area and dynamics if balance is to be more than merely gravitational.

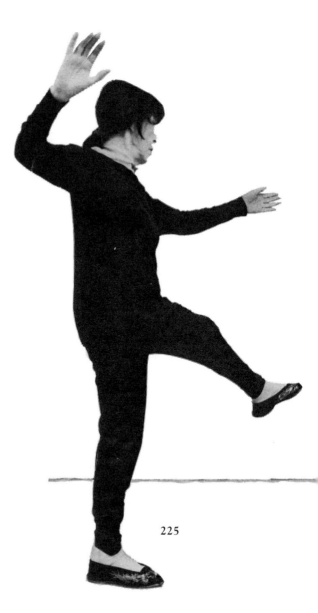

225

When the various parts of the body are properly aligned according to the needs of the structure, the result will be without strain, with no extraneous effort and false pressure and will therefore be in absolute balance. One of the aims of t'ai-chi ch'üan is to know how the body 'works' and so be able, at all times and for any occupation, to hold and manipulate it correctly and with ease.

Balance is also mentally conditioned. The mind acts with differing degrees of effort, coordinated in the changing patterns. Mindless action destroys the moment of equilibrium. Mind helps to produce stability and at the same time reflects it by being itself stable and clear. Attention, awareness, consciousness contribute to the dynamic interplay of action. Mind adds not only a superior ability to function, but also a heightened perceptiveness and acute discernment of the interweaving subtle ingredients that make balance absolute.

Since motion, regulated by space and time, is constant, the word perpetual cannot be used superfluously or superficially. When gravitational balance is maintained absolutely, we do indeed have perpetual motion in absolute balance—or can we say perpetual balance in absolute motion?

There are still more elements to the quality of absolute balance in addition to position, form, movement and dynamics. The following are aspects of the structure significant to the concept of absolute balance: (1) The 108 Forms and 108 Transitions in alternating balance throughout; (2) the balanced qualities of the different Forms—void (*Hsü*) and full (*Shih*); (3) the relationship of simple and complex Transitions; (4) the changing energies of both mind and body; (5) the flowing connectiveness of all action, making an ending a new beginning, physically and mentally.

The concept of absoluteness of t'ai-chi ch'üan can be compared to the totality of space-time-energy elements of the planets rotating around the sun—a composition of multiplicity in motion, of ordered diversity, making a supreme unity.

The total exercise is a balance of the active beginning (Transition-yang) and the quiet conclusion of the final moment (Form-yin), the body being in equilibrium and the mind in equanimity.


## 7. The Play of Breathing: Natural and Controlled

In the course of the t'ai-chi ch'üan journey we do not interfere with the usual everyday manner of breathing. The harmoniously balanced structure with its dynamic interplay of Yin-Yang forces conforms to the rhythm and timing of the natural breathing process.

The alternating physiological changes of the body-form acting like a bellows, function with and take care of inhalation and exhalation—which come and go so naturally that breathing does not seem to exist. Even at the conclusion of this long exercise breathing is regular, quiet and stable; often it has a slower tempo than at the start.

The depth of inhalation is not always the same. As in 'life', breathing levels change according to the type of activity, so in t'ai-chi ch'üan there are deeper and more shallow breaths responding to the way action and form move in relation to gravity, position and direction. The Stork Flaps its Wings (Form 7) is an example of a Form where the in-take of breath is full and deep as the figure rises from a curved, bent over and low position, to a straight vertical. A light exhalation is then made with a turn of a hand, which begins this yin Form.

In addition to the depth and lightness of breathing a natural way, there are different time-spans for patterns and breathing, both being simultaneous. Technically the varying breathing lengths are caused by slowed-up tempo, and by a long or short transition between Forms. Breathing changes are never mentally or emotionally instigated. Just as movement and change of form-gesture affect muscular dynamic changes, so the breathing process coincides with the shape and space of the action—and most importantly, without ever speeding up the rate of the heart beat.

The plan of the structure, mirroring nature's way, makes breathing so easy that the beginning student, of no matter what temperament, is unaware of breathing. The basic t'ai-chi ch'üan principle that mind must be centered on the activity contributes decidely to the fact that breathing goes and comes unnoticed.

As described, this natural breathing moves of itself and adjusts to the changing conditions of movement. Just as the circulatory system, regulating itself, is stimulated and improved by diverse t'ai-chi ch'üan activity, so the breathing process is helped and made more secure by the consciously applied physical activity. Both instinctive systems respond to the scientifically created activity made more efficient by the ever present use of the mind. T'ai-chi ch'üan fortifies health by increasing the ability of the cardiovascular system to function smoothly.

Controlled breathing is an advanced method for self-development. This technique is a difficult one to do with the constantly changing complex structure. It therefore must be attempted only when one has become exceedingly proficient in guiding body and mind so harmoniously that the action has become "second nature". Instead of keeping the attention on the process of the patterns and Forms as is done with natural breathing, in the controlled method, concentration is centered on the *breathing* activity— knowing *where* the breath is at all times in the movement of the changes.

Fundamentally, natural breathing variations continue within the controlled and conscious way. In the latter breathing is, on the whole, done in *slower* time. For instance, when a Transition in natural breathing style requires two 'in and out' breaths, the same pattern will be done with *one* 'in and out' breath in the controlled.

Controlled breathing does not imply inhibition or artificiality. The laws of nature are being effectively obeyed, with keen observation of how the body functions in terms of the multi-relationships and complexities of physiological behavior.

This deeply conscious control of breathing should be attempted only when one is 'relatively' perfect in rendering Form, Transition, space and tempo; to do it prematurely is dangerous. As a caution, the practitioner should note whether he or she (1) has excellent coordination in moving from one place to another; (2) experiences the subtleties of yin-yang dynamics to sustain the flowing continuity, (3) can retain the basic tempo with one part of the body while another part moves more slowly, (4) feels the yin aspect of the Form, and (5) masters, among other elements, the curvilinear directions of the shapes and shades of structure. When these aspects are 'engrained' in mind and body, controlled breathing will have become a 'natural'.

The *Shin-San Shih Hsing-Kung Hsin Chieh* (Chapter 5 above) warns: "Too much preoccupation with the breath, makes one clumsy. The appearance of 'lack of breath' is real strength".

## 8. *The Mind Connection*

The thought of mind activity has been emphasized throughout these pages as a motivating force which commands the body's actions; as a self-improving power; as a 'comforting' entity which creates equanimity.

Although the structure is basically mind-directed, the organization of body forms has within it the power to animate the mind. Significantly, mind and structure play double roles—in acting with and reacting to each other. Mind can be seen in another light—that as a directing element it can be a receiving one. It can be stirred to stay with the body, connected to the structured way which had been created to coordinate body and mind.

The technical means by which mind is helped to remain with the action, and by which it is kept alert to respond to changes and prevented from evaporating, and the physical means which are 'mindful' of the intrinsicality of effort, include the following elements, all pertinent to the way of structure.

1. Coordination—the root of the integration of the constant motion and the changing Forms, challenges the mind's attention.
2. Length of the exercise—gives mind 'holding' power, to persevere and to remain calm and stable.
3. Diversity of subtle changes—keeps mind alert and attentive.
4. Repetitions—make mind aware of the 'inattention' of the body which will reverse into familiar patterns automatically.

5. Surprise sequences—shocks to force mind to use more effort (yang) to attend.
6. Differences in slowed-up tempi—sharpen mind in coordinating and in connecting form with time in space.
7. Dynamic interchange—keeps mind on appreciation of gravitational and structural balances.
8. Intricacies of shape and movement—sharpen sensitivity to the aesthetic principle of form and function.
9. Physiological changes—alert mind's attention to the body experience of the harmony of joint-muscle movement.
10. Simple and complex transitions—give mind awareness of its own (yin) 'rest' and (yang) effort.
11. Everchanging direction—makes mind able to relate to repeated Forms differently.
12. Stillness in activity—sensitizes mind to the perception of the existence of the quiet centered in the action.

Mind being stimulated and mind-stimulating activities are inseparable, since the 'Methods' for both are organically integrated. We can say the mind functions 'acrobatically' in being able to separate and interlock the multiple tasks of the exercise; in being able to conceive and perceive; and in being able, amid the unceasing changingness of all things, to create "oneness" by being centered and so to produce peace of mind.

## 9. The Substance of Containment

Throughout the execution of the exercise, a state of containment has been developing gradually. It is sensed substantially at the completion of all movement, when the body is still, when mind seems not to exist and the body is not felt. There is, however, deep within the system a stirring awareness of a special and glowing aliveness which pervades the entire being.

Containment differs radically from the feeling of contentment in which the mental and physical body become extremely relaxed and complacent; this induces an agreeable self-satisfying emotion of not wanting, and not needing or caring to do anything in the wide world.

Containment never produces a feeling of being gravity-bound but is instead an airy and bouyant sensation as if one could rise and float as lightly as a balloon. Alertly unself-conscious, containment contains a sense of supreme consciousness which gives promise of further insights into oneself.

The substance of form-structure and of balanced interaction of dynamics of movement; of unceasing mind awareness of yin-yang diversities; of the tangible and intangible process of action; of the comprehension of the evolving structure as it takes place over a specific period of time—all is substance which, transformed, becomes containment, and which when truly experienced seems to have come as if by itself.

The attention at the concluding moment of t'ai-chi ch'üan is not the same as it was at the beginning, when the mind is active. Attention at the end is quiet, settled on the experience of wholeness. All practitioners of t'ai-chi ch'üan at any stage of proficiency, are sensitive to the contained heart-mind-body equality when the exercise is completed. T'ai-chi ch'üan transcends the limitations of the player, who is led by "the mysterious potency" of its structure.

Meaning saturates the Method; Method envelops the Meaning. From both spring peacefulness and contained vitality. The t'ai-chi ch'üan experience, that of mind-body harmony, embraces, without effort, the spirit of containment.

## CHAPTER 9

# The Art of the Science of T'ai-Chi Ch'üan: A Summary

In the science of t'ai-chi ch'üan lies the definite knowledge of how man can best regulate himself in all aspects of living—physically, emotionally, mentally. In the art of t'ai-chi ch'üan lies the process that produces a state of harmonious well-being and, with this, the realization that man can achieve and experience a unique sense of emotional and mental integration.

The science and the art are inseparable and are experienced simultaneously. Both function through a technique which is dominated by a *way*, a textured way of moving that determines the effect of this multifaceted composition. This way is embedded in the very nature of its aims (its science), and it is the cause of the essential inner experience and the outer expression (its art).

This Exercise-Art, the antithesis of the accidental, the unpremeditated, the blindly inspirational, is composed, ordered, figured out, and developed according to theory, thought, philosophy, science, mathematics, and the laws of nature.

The concrete material of this physical exercise correlates all of man's faculties as he puts his body into action, his mind into awareness, and his spirit into serenity. Compose the body and the mind is calmed; settle the mind and the emotions are composed. The thought, the feeling, the action—each can be the root, the link, the cause, and the effect. Whichever the way, the result is a balance of the vital energy of body and mind.

Although this composition is not an original for anyone, the participator, in reenacting the structure, creates it anew, so to speak, and is transformed by it. He himself becomes the work of art in the doing of it. Comprehension of what he is doing, and the awareness of what it is, makes it possible for him to achieve the harmony of physical security, emotional ease, mental poise, and what is essential to the spirit of t'ai-chi ch'üan, to experience its aesthetic quality.

It is the science of its structure based on the natural laws of body-behavior and action that produces the power of sustained good health. It is the art that creates the heart-mind (in Chinese—*hsin*) ease, its containment (emotional), and contentment (aesthetic).

With t'ai-chi ch'üan it is the doer, the performer of this masterpiece, who reacts to the art of this art at the same time as he becomes the art, as he lives it in space and from moment to moment. Observers are not needed for the aesthetic completion of this work of art. They may become engrossed by it and may detect its artistic nature, and although they may (possibly) understand it, they cannot *feel* its intrinsic nature, which is part of its art. Because the onlookers cannot benefit from the *function* of its form, they cannot have the true aesthetic experience.

When I first saw t'ai-chi ch'üan being practiced in the T'ai Miao Park in Peking, the impact on me was one of such unusual power that I knew it could not be measured by any already learned standards, however profound.

The beauty of the flow of movement seemingly effortless, the harmonious designs of the interlacing forms, and the calm composition as balanced as the horizon made me feel that the doer was experiencing from the process of action something—a sense of being—which could not be projected outward to affect the observer similarly; that what I was experiencing was an elementary awareness of its art-nature, not the full aesthetic nature of its art, which came from the doing and not from the seeing, as I was to discover from later experiences.

We have an art when the harmonious blending of form and function arouses a special feeling in the observer as in the Fine Arts, and, as I believe, when it produces a state of being in the doer, as in t'ai-chi ch'üan.

Art, without purpose or direction, without motivation for the form, generally results in being mechanically formal. Subject matter, no matter how important, will never alone make an art art worthy; it must be significantly expressed in terms of the art medium. In t'ai-chi ch'üan form and function are so totally integrated that function functions through the form, and form reveals and becomes the function. Complete synthesis produces what I call a fourth dimension, the aesthetic content. T'ai-chi ch'üan is an art for the one who enacts it; for the observer, it produces a state of sympathetic awareness of an art and arouses, empathetically, a state of repose.

The way of the movement, the body technique, and the space design and body configurations are absolutely the consequence of the goals and benefits to be derived from performing the complete exercise daily. There is no vagueness about the principles for self-development. To improve the body's health, physical skill, and stamina is to increase the possibility for longer life. The ability to concentrate and coordinate and to deepen mental perceptivity and alertness produces quicker reflexes, awareness, observation, and control, and therefore greater harmony of thought and action. Coordination of mind and body is conducive to calmness, without which no one can be considered truly healthy. Such harmony and the exploration of qualities deep in man not yet awakened—these are the concepts which had inspired various Chinese philosophers to devote their lives to the creation of an exercise art which would realize these goals.

Substance of this movement-art is in the Form: how it comes into being; how it is completed; how it changes and becomes another Form.

Substance is in the action: it is the working relationship between muscles and joints; it is the transformation of a Transition to a Form; it is the texture (yin-yang) of the movement. This substance is "controlled yet airy in appearance"; it has "the stillness of a mountain and the agility of a river"; it contains the spirit of the concentrated alertness of "a cat waiting to catch a mouse"; and it has the form in potential speed of "a hawk trying to snatch a rabbit." The collective aspect of substance contributes to the fine art of this exercise art.

Form forms the space; time shapes the patterns; and space times the Forms. The ingredients of shape, space, time (tempo), pattern, direction, and substance are factors continually at play in such impeccable relationships that, (1) the body, internally and externally, is in perfect equilibrium; (2) the yin-yang elements are proportionately related; (3) unity in every active moment is apparent despite the complexity of changes. It is a world of changing unities. (see Chapter 7.)

The discipline of making the mind stay with one is an intrinsic part of the structure of this exercise. It can never be walked through; it must be lived through each time. This develops a mental alertness that becomes part of every day living and working. With true awareness which gives security, self-consciousness, which is emotional ill-ease, will *never* intrude on the consciousness.

What happens in space is never accidental nor arbitrary, mainly because man's physiological structure determines the design, i.e., that every movement affects the shape of the space. Accurately made space directions will help to improve the body's form by way of joint articulations. Correctly made body positions will take place in the designated areas. Structure can be manipulated by space placement; space can adjust the forms. If a stance is incorrect because of the improper body position, i.e., hips thrust out in back forcing the leg and spine alignment to be wrong, the change of movement in space will not work. If the spatial design is wrong, i.e., too widely or narrowly spaced, the body will not be able to move correctly into the next specific design. The body checks the space and the space the body's unity. To understand this is to see the total unification of inner and outer structures, the interfusion of science of the body and the art of its use in space, the juxtaposition of the tangible and intangible, and the harmony of self in action in relation to static environment.

The observer responds agreeably to the manifest inevitability of movement sequences—a coming out in the right place at the right time; this is harmony of space and form. The observer does not have to wait for a resolution of a series of movements and a climax of ideas, because the idea exists at every moving moment, visibly. For the doer, the accumulation of these moments over a 22-25 minute period is another matter and of greatest significance, since the most valuable effect of t'ai-chi ch'üan lies in its length, just as eating the whole apple is more salutary for the body's needs than a single bite, as the greater benefits are contained in and attained from the accumulation of the Forms, although each unit is composed of the ingredients of the whole.

The floor pattern the feet traverse is as exact as a mathematical equation (see foot chart). The enclosing shape is that of a rectangle, the side to side (east and west) width being fourteen footsteps long, each individual's foot size, not the standard measurement, determining the distance. The front to back (north and south) length is seven footsteps long. The east-west axis line comes between the second and third footstep. The starting *and* the finishing space is at the same point, being at the fourth step in from the right (east) with the toes touching the axis line. It must be said here that the off center floor placement is typical for *all* postures. A symmetrical position is fairly static and coming as it does away from a centered point, its immobile effect is diminished, while its restful effects are augmented. The awareness of space is three dimensional; the four upper and four lower diagonal corners, as angled from the torso itself, are important in respect to body design and space structure. Every person recognizes the limits of his own seven by fourteen rectangle, even when the exercise is done out-of-doors as is generally done in China. (See page 168).

It can be seen that such complexity of direction is more than moving the feet along a path, but this directional aspect is absolutely simple compared to the multitude of changes the body is capable of even in that confined space. And these changes and variations, though complex, are *not* uncalculated— they have been chosen, regulated, selected, devised by *plan* which adheres to the intent (as function) and to the essential principles (as form).

Combined meaningfully as they are (in every unit of action) with every angle of the 360 degree circle, and with every structural requirement of body in space scrupulously considered, it can be appreciated how scientifically profound and artfully astute were the philosophic creators of t'ai-chi ch'üan— the more so because nothing is abstracted from Meaning, although the Method is objective and universal.

The textured way of movement is by far the most important technique to carry out specific goals. Aesthetically, this moving way is the most apparent of all the techniques and has the greatest effect on the onlooker and it is the most difficult to achieve. This way is the continuity in movement— which builds up endurance; it is the subtlety of moving the joints (to link up form)—which develops keen perceptivity; it is the never-stopping, endless flow which increases control; it is itself calm, evokes calmness—which improves concentration.

The way of smoothly sustained movement is described (in the *T'ai-Chi Ch'üan* Canon, fifteenth century) as resembling "the even control (in pulling) required to draw out the silk thread from a cocoon": to pull jerkily would break the thread; to pull too lightly is ineffectual. To achieve the correct technique, the mind must be centered and control the activity. The accomplishment of mind-body unity creates a sense of tranquility which, inwardly felt, is radiated outward.

The way of holding the muscles comes from the structure itself, just as carrying a heavy or light load demands a different degree of energy expended. In t'ai-chi ch'üan all changes of intensities are never made visibly, never externalized. This is an intrinsic exercise: changes of force result from the designs and Forms themselves, so that muscular variations are built-in, therefore invisible (but, of course, greatly felt). What makes this concealed effort possible is the way the movements move into each other through joint action, by the balance of the structural sequences as they relate to space, and by the fact that the alternation of yin and yang dynamics is microscopically gradual, giving time to the body to adjust itself intrinsically to the changing forms.

The way of the formation of the Forms and Transitions is circular—the "going" is curvi-form, as arc, spiral, loop, oval, crescent, parabola, etc., a circle or any part thereof. There are, according to my way of thinking, two classes of curve: the natural physical way, and the designed, created, curvilinear motion (page 171).

The designed curve is a creative extension of the physiological fact, and a necessary addition since the main purpose of this exercise is to augment the natural condition of body and mind, far beyond the things we were born with. Because of our very complexity, the nature of the circular action must correspondingly be extended far above the natural, yet, as can be seen, always working with, in turn with, the natural.

From the fact that the beginning Form and the ending Form are at the same place, we can perceive the architectural space to be in the form of a circle, with the diagonal directions to be considered as segments, a circle within a rectangle. Our rectangular (so to speak) body describes spatial circles at every turn, low or high, right or left, rectangle within a circle.

Structurally speaking, the curve is everywhere: in the natural turn of a wrist and in the designed half-circle of an arm gesture (Figure 226).

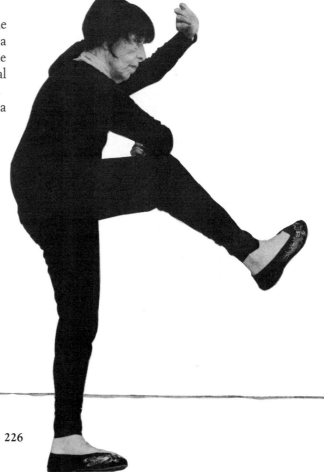

226

A complex combination of a parabolic curve of an arm, timed with a half turn of a wrist, as the head turns and dips, with the leg making a hooklike pattern, this is typical of the variety of design and curve that appears throughout the exercise. And not to lose sight of its function— such action develops coordination and stability, awareness and perception of the subtle.(Figure 227)

The curve shades action and stillness from the obvious actions to the most delicate refinements, like the movements of a wave propelling itself into, and therefore making, another wave. Ability to balance at every conceivable moment is made possible by the curved-way action. The circular way prevents expenditure of energy and reserves strength to be used only when needed. In the process of doing the exercise the expended moment of finality, like "the shooting or letting-go of the arrow," is never part of the action. Rather, the body feeling is like that of the stretching of the bow, always ready to take off, alive, poised, concentrated and aware and reserved, ready for the final blow. The curved way with its wave-like, to and fro, give and take dynamics contributes to the resilient activity of muscles, which method gives the body elasticity and pliability.

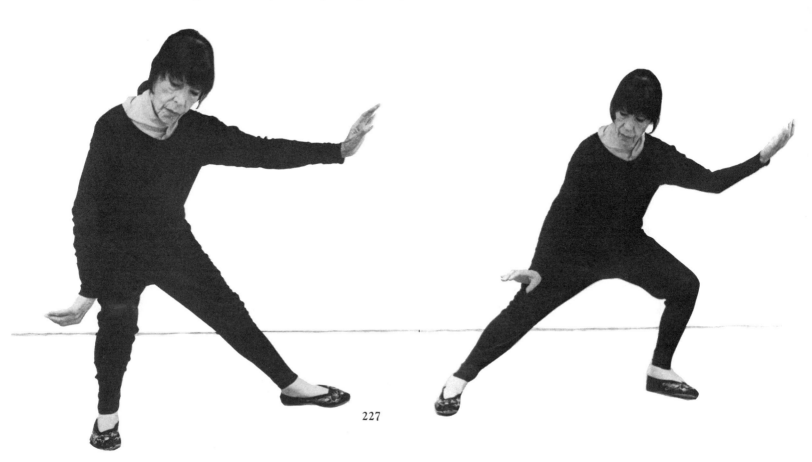

227

A circle embraces one with security, and distils containment. The concept of the circle creates stillness and calmness. And contained as the multiple complexities are within it, the result is a balance of the two forces of activity and stillness.

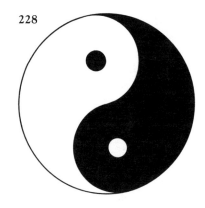

The T'ai-chi shape symbolizes the containment of the continuous flow of energy which, according to universal principles, is of two kinds, the yin and the yang. These two opposite forces, to cite some examples, like ebb and flow, diastole-systole, negative-positive, stillness-movement, female-male, backward-forward, moon-sun, earth-heaven, etc., balance and partner each other, never in opposition, but always as complements; the indisputable fact is that we can not and do not have one without the other. In this T'ai-chi symbol, the inference is that each, containing as it does a touch of the other (yin in yang, yang in yin), evolves into and dissolves from the other with complete and irrefutable consistency, based as it is on the fact that there is nothing without change in the universe (Figure 228).

This point of view explains and is reflected both in the palette, the muscle-tone coloration in movement-technique, and in the changing formations of the structure. The palette is limited by the natural organic process of energy changes required by the structural forms. This is the t'ai-chi ch'üan way. The lightest tone is light to that degree of tension which keeps the body in control and active. In the entire exercise there is never any relaxed position (succumbing to gravity) as, for instance, a loose head or dropped hand on an outstretched arm would be. Every movement is contemplated, directed, and controlled. The strongest muscular tension results from intrinsic form and not from subjective extraneous manipulation, such as *tensing* the fist to exhibit strength. The body is always capable of *more* strength than it shows or ever uses. But the extent of the dynamics is nevertheless very great indeed, as the movement moves from the lightest tone of a simple gesture to very complicated positions demanding great inner force to make and hold them. Because of such intrinsic restraints, and because the circular way dominates the shape-form, the external appearance of all the action seems effortless and weightless.

In a work of art, not only must all the components be there but, what is most important, their order and arrangement must be profoundly considered to achieve the art—the artistic and the desired effect. In t'ai-chi ch'üan the Forms, progressing and evolving through a complex path of structure, tempo, dynamics accomplish their goals by the collective force of selected ingredients (science) and their compositional arrangement (art), finally arrived at by those Chinese philosophers who had knowledge of the life of nature and the nature of life.

Though t'ai-chi ch'üan is an arranged structure, it is no stereotype. Just as the personal foot-size regulates the traversed distance of the floor area, so does the individual's body proportions determine the balance of the configurations made with torso, arms, and legs around itself. But the patterned movements themselves are mathematically directed in external terms, as in the angled degree in which the figure turns in any of the eight directions, in the placement of the foot in 45°, 90°, or 135° angles, etc. The composition itself is exactly determined and designed, as to where the arms, legs, knees, head, etc., are to be moved; but the individual's physiology will subtly determine the degree of the body curve and knee-bend action, or the height of a raised leg. However, the balanced result in each and every person must be the same: the same, let us say, as a circle is a circle whether it is small or large. In the Forms and their formings, the process is quite complicated since each moment of moving involves tempo, space, structure, *yin-yang* dynamics, balance, stillness, and activity, which make the totality.

Figure 229 illustrates the various points in the above paragraph. In the Single Whip Form, the heels are separated from each other by the length of two paces, which space differs for people with different foot sizes. The depth to which the knees bend depends on personal ability and flexibility, too; but the body attitude is the same for all—the knees must be in line with the toes, the torso and waist must be in correct position, the toes must point to the stipulated compass angles, and the entire direction of the Form must be exact in terms of outer space. This is an example of the personal self being disciplined objectively. Because of the logic of our common organic structure, such objective discipline does not violate our personalities. And because of our 'individualistic' natures there is never to be seen any chorus-like uniformity. Rather, through the regulated order and perfection of the moving postures, the individual's capacities, sensibilities, and abilities are heightened and sensitized.

The elements of structure in any single pattern are balanced, in terms of gravity, dynamics, space, and form; all are resolved proportionately in minute measurements and in exact ratio, so that at every moment peaceful harmony is felt and conveyed.

What happens in the distribution of size and weight, strength and lightness is clear when we take as an example a pound of feathers, which takes a large space, and balance it with a pound of iron, which takes up a small space. In t'ai-chi ch'üan when a leg design is light (*Hsü*—void), the space covered is greater than its balancing counterpart which is compact (*Shih*—solid), and the rest of the body will be patterned with varying degrees of lightness and strength, making complete unity.

In Hand Strums the Lute, Figure 230, the right leg with bent knee is solid, carrying most of the weight, and the left leg, outstretched, rests lightly on the heel, covering as much ground as the length of leg permits. The right arm with palm turned outward (yang) is strongly centered halfway toward the chest, and the left arm with palm inward (yin) is lightly placed outside of right so that fingers reach right wrist. The larger space of light left arm balances the smaller space of the stronger right arm, as do the legs: the light left covers a large space and the strong right is in small body space.

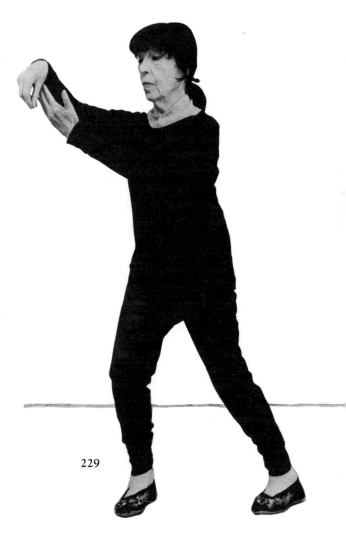

229

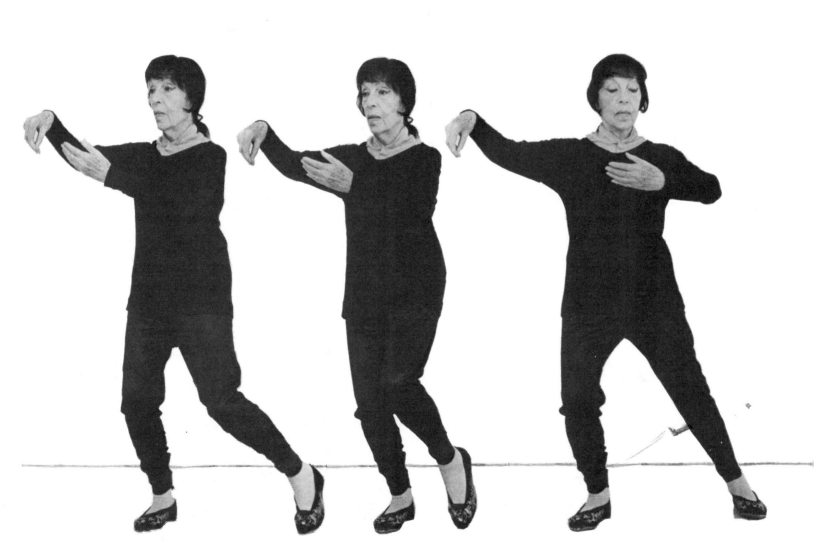

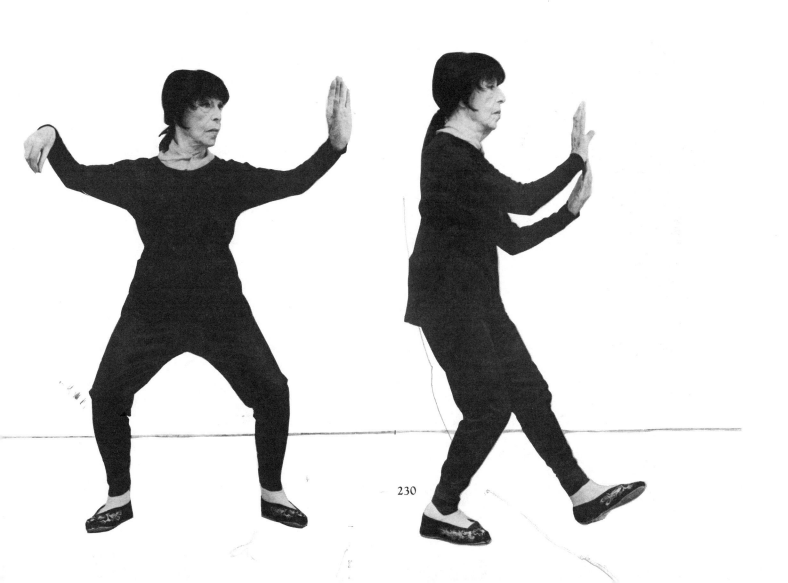

So impeccably balanced is each moving Form that "a single feather added to one's body and a false movement would destroy the balance." Placing the left hand, for instance (in the above figure), inside the right hand space would feel as awkward as hearing a wrong note struck in a familiar phrase. The measure of the changing weight balances the power and makes the power of balance: power is not force; it is the ability to control.

Every Form and Transition can be analyzed, each with its own sum of balances. The flow of movement is also securely balanced at each fractional second. As mentioned earlier, the dynamics cannot be seen because of their intrinsic nature. In the interweaving and dovetailing of pattern into pattern, the proportion of space to space is never *not* right. Arrangement and dynamics, space-size and the textured way, are correlated much in the same way as a colorist would harmonize the pale or brilliant, the dark or light hue in respect to space and juxtaposition in organizing his canvas to express his ideas.

In t'ai-chi ch'üan, however, since it is a moving canvas, the Transitions, transmitted like the perpetual flow of a river, displace and alter each situation so skillfully that depth and space, framework and Form, appear and disappear with singular ease. With such a Method, the mind is always intrigued, the power of the action stabilized, and the element of calmness increased.

The greater the balance, the lighter is the look. The more fluid the Transitions, the less visible is the technique, which in turn is then more proficient. Seen is the design, the action, the activity of structural and directional changes in relation to each other and to a "still part", i.e., that part of the body which does not change its position. Without a point of reference, a point of contrast, so much activity as has been described could become excessive and produce restlessness, in terms of t'ai-chi ch'üan principles.

In the course of changing (with a few exceptions), some part of the body is momentarily still. I analyze *stillness* as being of three kinds: (1) as related both to body and space; (2) as related to space; (3) as related to body. The first is most easily seen and done. A stance is taken and legs and torso remain still while the arms, head, fingers move. This is activity taking place in an obviously held position. Here we have control and rest at the same time. (Fig 231)

Second, stillness in relation to space means that one part of the body is kept in the same geometric relationship to space despite movement in the rest of the body. In the Form where the left leg is sidewards and the left arm is parallel to the floor, the left arm will remain in this parallel-space position all the time, while the left and right knees bend, thus lowering the torso and while the torso turns to face east. (Fig 232)

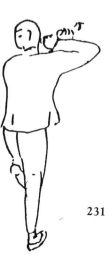

231

Third, stillness in relation to body means that a particular part does not move from its position in relation to the body, while its geometric place in space is being changed by movement in *another* part of the body. In The Stork Flaps Its Wings, the right arm, circled around the head, remains fixed in this position while the torso bends, twists, and rises (Fig. 233).

The still or suspended movement forms an aspect of space design that demands a new control. The ability to isolate and control any part of the body in its context with the planned form is another unique way to elevate the standard of coordination in both body and mind. From a purely physical standpoint, such non-action as in the paragraph above, third, gives more power to resist the pull of gravity. In the paragraphs above, second and third, we have examples of sets of muscles exercised, not by themselves moving but by action in a connected part, like that of moving the torso and shoulders around to each side while keeping the head still, to exercise the neck muscles.

Visually and physically, the design of action contrasted with a still motif becomes more and more complex, especially when gestures are moved in opposition. Add to this the fact of subtle tempo variations and the possibility for multiple sub-relationships of themes increases enormously.

Space form determines tempo, and the tempo shapes the space. The original and basic tempo, decided upon by the opening gesture, is always present, being carried by some part of the moving body at all times. This basic tempo controls the Form and dominates the movement in space. But within this basic tempo are slower tempi of varying slownesses.

To illustrate tempo and Form synchronization, take the familiar minute and second hands of a clock, both of which arrive at their destined moment together, making a unity of sixty seconds and one minute. This action is smooth, regular, precise. In the execution of certain Forms, a similar but more complicated synthesis takes place, because some part of the body may be moving with different tempi.

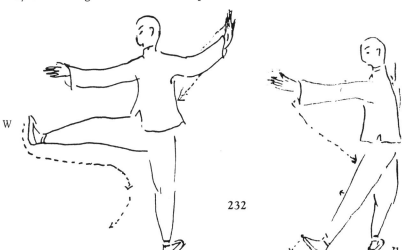

232

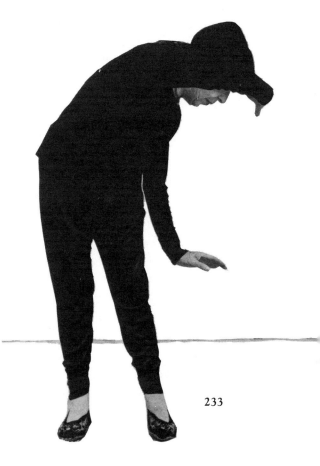

233

Since each Form is a synchronized moment, it is inferred that all parts of the body have to arrive at their appointed places at the same moment. Some parts will have had to move over large or small areas, therefore taking different time periods to culminate the Form simultaneously. The rule is that the basic tempo is maintained by the part moving in the largest space. The tempo used in the smaller spaces is always slowed down, the degree of slowness depending on the relative distances, as, for example, an arm moving in a quarter circle will have to slow down by half the tempo taken by an arm making a half circle, if they are to meet at the same place, together.

From a position where the body and legs are still, the crossed hands must move to meet at the left ear; the right arm makes a large circle at the same time that the left makes a short arc to reach the place. The right arm maintains the basic tempo, while the left moves more than twice as slowly. This is a broad example of tempo differences. When areas have less differentiation, the degrees of tempo changes are delicate indeed. The orchestration of arms, legs, torso, head, turning, lowering and lifting, going forward and backward, demands a deep perception of time as well as structure. The proportions of the flowing pictures must be controlled with concentration and patience. The feeling of calm comes from accuracy, and mental enrichment comes from the varying complexities. The greater the perfection of synchronization the more the enjoyment, the more profound the perception, the richer the experience of the art.

The wonder of t'ai-chi ch'üan is the lack of clock-time feeling despite such specific delineations of time and space. The objective feeling of a vacuum of time arises from the unending continuity of the moving process, from the "seamlessness" of the interlacing forms, and especially from the constancy of balance—the composite order of all which produces a state of weightlessness in the body (and of no-limit to the psyche).

The composition as a whole is comprehended and appreciated only after all the individual units which are small totalities have been learned in unaltered sequence. It is the reverse of how we generally come to understand a picture, where first we look for the dominating structure or the central theme, after which we analyze the detailed elements. In t'ai-chi ch'üan, because each idea-unit is complete in itself and leads with consistency into another unit, perception grows with the experience of relating them to each other. It is when the small total Forms are comprehended that the larger masses which embrace them can be recognized as being made up of the same forces, but fashioned less obviously and more ingeniously. Consciousness of the greater structures increases the aesthetic appreciation of the scientific whole.

The exercise is divided into six series, each quite individual in character, and differing as to: spatial planning and the main lines of direction (advancing in Series I, and retreating in Series II); the demands made on energy for balancing (Series III); the levels of coordination and concentration (in Series

IV); the psychological device of using repeated themes (in Series V); the introduction of new themes until the very last moment of action to keep attention and interest from flagging (in Series VI). Each section has its unique group of Forms, stimulating the mind and using the body in special ways.

What is seen and felt in the microcosm is appreciated and experienced in the macrocosm on a large scale and in different proportions: alternation of opposite forces like bending-straightening, forward-backward, opening-closing, in-out, up-down, powerful-easy, complex-simple, etc.; changing weight dynamics; variety in Form and tempo; ebb and flow in movement sensation; variations in design so that the body never tires. The facts of balance and of continuous movement are innate, as is the never-ending, never-ceasing flow, so that the division between any two series (just as between the Forms) is never visible.

Even with such a variegated process of multiple patterns within Forms, and Forms within Series, there is never a touch of superfluity in pattern, design, movement; no unneeded gesture, no decoration ever appears. Even in the most strenuous of positions, no superfluous demands are made upon the body. With the technique of learning to "lift a pound of energy," all movements are true to use, consistent, never awkward, therefore beautiful.

The most minute turn of every gesture is selected, every action is chosen and combined according to the intrinsic laws of how the body functions best, and to the limitations set by the long-time objectives based on mental equanimity. It is inevitable that artistry should grow out of such implicit rightness. We can say that t'ai-chi ch'üan is a marvelous example of beauty and use and becomes a truthful experience when practiced.

Although the machinery of the human body is fantastically complicated and its structured action equally so, the coordinated resultant look in practicing is innocent, i.e., harmonious, balanced, beautiful. The elasticity of the line of action, with its sensitive fluctuations of yin and yang and its intermeshing circlings, makes the body use itself, not only not superfluously, but economically. Again we can take the working of a clock as an example and compare our structure to it, since rightness comes out of need, no matter how complicated the means.

The body is ultimately at its best when it is not felt. The painful back, the strained neck and shoulders make us know disagreeably the presence of those parts. Like a bridge which appears light because the forces and stresses of its alignment are so mathematically correct and balanced, so the human being feels light and appears so when muscles and joints behave correctly, in tune with each other. And when we are not conscious of the body—meaning in the absence of irregularities—then the emotions are most neutral and, paradoxically, most pleasant, meaning the presence of harmony; well-being is, then, conscious, and vitality is at its maximum. Through its extraordinary discipline, t'ai-chi ch'üan helps each person to discover and create a set of balances for the living of life.

In any work of art we expect to see a consistency in content, substance, and values. But even more, we expect to have continuing gratification and pleasure from a work that is an art and from which we expect to experience new profundities.

With t'ai-chi ch'üan, the more familiarity, the deeper its aspects, the richer its possibilities. To do it is to discover it anew, and to discover it is to penetrate its layers. No one submits himself to this exercise, as one does to a medicine. The spirit and the will power must be willing. But then, according to my experience, t'ai-chi ch'üan is so artisically and emotionally persuasive that even the raw and ignorant beginner finds a new will, a wish to do it, and pursue it.

In t'ai-chi ch'üan, the means is an end in itself. But also, like its philosophy, it is a beginning, a means for some other end, other purpose. It is a beginning in its application for a way in the conduct of life and work.

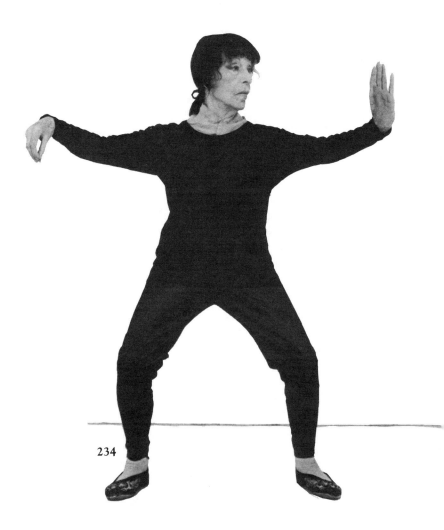

234

# Part Four:

*The Life of T'ai-Chi Ch'üan*

The inner vitality awakened by the everyday process of 'playing' (the literal translation of the Chinese word for practice) t'ai-chi ch'üan, stimulates the sensibilities to move in many paths of creativity. Like the branches of a tree which spread out in profusion, and yet because of their nature never go beyond the shape and form of the particular species, so the branches of the mind in no matter what flight of thought—practical, poetic, philosophical, psychological, and spiritual—are rooted in, and stay within the scope of, the life-force principles of t'ai-chi ch'üan.

Each unique aspect can be individually highlighted without fragmenting the totality. Counterexchange of the forces of mind-body-thought-feeling-action arouses deep interest in the life of the Meaning's Method and the Method's Meaning; and is the source of equanimity and the resource for creative fulfillment.

### An Air of Innocence

T'ai-chi ch'üan is an innocent-looking exercise. How can I use the word innocent for such a complex mind-body structure so philosophically and aesthetically profound, a structure which scientifically integrates space and form, and balances mental concentration with intricacies of body activity?

T'ai-chi ch'üan has the appearance of innocence because it is a continuum of flowing movement without any visible change of dynamics or tempo. Being in unfailing balance at all times, seemingly done without effort, adds to the look of ease, and therefore of innocence.

Since in t'ai-chi ch'üan no emotion colors the activity and no intellectualizing interferes with the making of the Forms, all action appears to grow 'naturally'. Anyone who experiences this exercise will always feel harmoniously 'just right', whether the person is mature or fairly new in the practice of this exercise-art.

I do not say it is an exercise *for* the innocent! It can be learned and done by the most sophisticated, by the naive, by the very ignorant. The exercise is simply enacted step by step with mind directing the manner of the movement and the matter of the patterns from which inevitably the participant will feel its harmonious objectivity.

T'ai-chi ch'üan is as 'innocent' as breathing—without which we cannot live and yet which is accepted so innocently and matter-of-factly. T'ai-chi ch'uan functions for all—naturally—because it is physically consistent with the laws of nature and, despite the coordinative complexities, it permits us to behave with the smooth and organic regularity of breathing. The unified balance of the whole makes the inner experience joyous and profound and produces *outwardly* the air of innocence.

Experiencing t'ai-chi ch'üan is more than a matter of balanced continuity, awareness and concentration. In the final analysis it is the greatness of the harmonious structure which vibrates with Meaning at every minute turn of the continuous action, and which insures the containment of innocence. Meaningfully planned from the first moment of action to the last moment of stillness, the structure puts the t'ai-chi ch'üan player into a state of receptivity. The compositional strength lies in the fact that one can be in complete control with calm concentration. The presence of the mind on the activity of the body, with the body alert to the activity of the mind, produces a look of unpremeditated thought.

Through the unity inherent in the many complexities, t'ai-chi ch'üan itself, not so innocently, creates a situation in which the participant cannot but project an air of artlessness—and so seems to *be* innocent.

## The Long Journey

T'ai-chi ch'üan takes you on a long journey. It is a long and smooth journey, a long and integrated journey; and above all, it is a profound journey. This slow-in-tempo journey can make time disappear. Sometimes it seems endless; or it may pass like a grand and monumental moment; but the journey itself will always move you with clock-time accuracy.

The journey is a complex one. The extraordinary paths of diverse movements are *never* not in balance and *never* without coherence and unity. No matter how subtle the action and intricate the maneuverings, the body-journey structures are physically at ease, and fall exactly into place in space and time, three-dimensionally sculptured.

As a profound journey, it is never abandoned by the mind, which not only directs the action but keeps you attentively aware and clear. The stumbling blocks of entangling emotions, distracting thoughts, and mental blackouts are erased as the journey progresses.

A hyperbole of balance, the journey functions securely in physical-emotional-mental dimensions.

T'ai-chi ch'üan, at each stage of its journey, fulfills the varied, promised goals directed toward a higher development of the self in terms of keener consciousness.

As a process of change and a changing process, nothing in the journey is trivial, nothing superfluous—from the most solid tangibles to the illusive intangibles; from the minute turn of a wrist to the augmented power of a stance; from a complex element culminating in a Form to the simplicity of an isolated gesture. Always throughout, the dynamic forces, light and strong (yin and yang) interweaving, are sensitively graded.

The journey creates many experiences and awakens awareness on many levels—physically, psychologically, intellectually, artistically, psychoanalytically, creatively. These aspects may overlap and be enmeshed one into the other or may be discerned separately. Always pleasurably interesting, every step of the way offers satisfaction for body and mind and for the spirit—even very early in the journey.

The greater the development, the more assured become the will and the willingness to repeat and continue the journey which inevitably becomes richer, more subtle, and more powerful. Although the journey in terms of self-development is endless, it has an ending in time, at which point the activity—the outer activity—ceases physically. All visible motion then has come to rest, but the journey within the self continues—consciousness of being calm, awareness of the presence of the quiet yet alert self with overtones of a newer vitality.

This journey's end becomes a new beginning, since every repetition contains the advanced and accumulated experiences of all that went before. We can respect the ever-increasing power of mind and body that each journey produces. Once the journey has been undertaken, the feeling that there is no end is extremely agreeable. As self-knowledge augments, it is intriguing to anticipate what could possibly happen as the *inner* journey progresses in depth and self-confidence.

When we say that this journey is "out of this world," we imply that the journey is more than could have possibly been perceived at the early stages of moving on the t'ai-chi ch'üan path. As one travels far enough, consciously enough, and *often* enough, the resulting unusual and contained sensation can be considered to *be* "out of this world".

Though it is important to get to the end of the journey for full effect, it nevertheless offers rewards at a succession of the 'smaller endings'. Each of the 108 Forms is a definite culmination of shorter sections and passages of varying time lengths. These are the many 'stations' of awareness on the way as one travels on toward the complete end.

During the journey, there is no feeling of division or separation. The totality—the sum of the 'small journeys'—brings one to a high level of accomplishment at every repetition of the entire journey.

T'ai-chi ch'üan, stronger than the self, helps one to endure the journey as it becomes progressively more profound.


## A Miracle of Movement


In an airy, sunlit studio at the Ohio University in Athens, I had just begun a demonstration of t'ai-chi ch'üan when, as someone later told me, a butterfly alighted on my shoulder and remained there for fully fifteen minutes—to the moment when I had to change the slow, flowing tempo to a flash of speedy action.

Lao Tzu wrote, "When the harmony of yin and yang is perfect, a bird can sit on your hand without being afraid." Perhaps the butterfly needs less impeccable harmony than a bird for it to stay in place on a moving human being. Nevertheless, it can be assumed that in terms of the smooth shifting of my weight from one intricate form to another, and most importantly because of the controlled stillness of my torso and shoulders, the yin and yang were harmonious enough to make the butterfly not afraid.

The even breathing process is so intimately related to the action, at all times, that even the sensitive butterfly was unaware of it, and what sent it on its separate way was the sudden change of pace.

Such an experience illustrates the intrinsic nature of t'ai-chi ch'üan movement—that it succeeds in giving one the power to remain quiet and fluidly continuous whatever the yin-yang dynamic variations are and no matter how the pattern relationships change. And it is to be especially noted that quick motions in t'ai-chi ch'üan do not change the breathing rhythm and that what startled the butterfly was the unexpected *action*. *Nothing* in t'ai-chi ch'üan disturbs the natural heartbeat or the breathing tempo. This is due not only to the *special* timing of movement to movement and space to space but also to the fact that all is done without emotional content.

The ability to balance the interweaving action smoothly, to look as if all were executed with equal lack of intensity, is indeed part of the movement miracle. Actually the dynamic variations even in a small area are always moving from 'empty' (slightly weighted) to 'solid' (strongly grounded) as well as from lightness to power—all done according to physiological requirements and gravity's demands. The structured movements of t'ai-chi ch'üan regulate the opposites so that all become harmonious. It will always feel miraculous that the perpetual interaction of space-dynamics can be so impeccably controlled.

The movement is a miracle of function in respect to the physiological clarity with which the complex Forms can be executed. One is in constant wonder that even the most minute and delicate of Transition, seemingly unseen, possess such "tangibility," the subtlety of which is both the cause and result of awakening awareness and deepening perception.

It is a moving miracle when t'ai-chi ch'üan structures can be applied so meticulously to our physiological and psychological selves that body stamina and mind ease are simultaneously developed.

The flow of movement is a miracle of balance—every unit of Form, every Transition being spatially and dynamically adjusted with mathematical exactitude to prevent the force of gravity from throwing one off one's 'center', physically and mentally.

The way of t'ai-chi ch'üan is the essence of grace. Being smooth, even, light, and flowing would, it seems, be enough for a technique to be termed graceful, but the grace in t'ai-chi ch'üan evolves from the complex intricacies both of the Way and the Movements which weave their curvilinear paths in inevitable harmony with space and time—a universal grace.

This essential grace, and with it dignity, permeates the self when the mind is present (as it must be) with the action. The atmosphere created from mind-body grace is as restful and secure as is the calm curve of the horizon and as contained as the arc of the sky.

No less a miracle is the fact that the total personality is always engaged with the process of the moving activity. No matter what the technical concerns are, no matter where the emphasis lies, and no matter how the mind moves, the self sustains a feeling of wholeness. Even the merest beginner in this complex art experiences at moments this intrinsic wholeness and is led by such awareness to stay with the 'long journey' and move toward more profound and long-lasting perceptions.

## The Moving Spirit

As we move along in flowing style through the forms of t'ai-chi ch'üan, a special sensation is unfailingly present—a pleasant feeling of repose that seems to make a unit of body, mind, and emotion. This feeling-sensation which coexists with and corresponds to the activity that is taking place can be named "The Moving Spirit."

The simultaneity of *moving* and *spirit* is so uniquely achieved in this exercise-art that we need hardly ask whether it is the spirit that moves or whether it is the movement which gives rise to the spirit. One blended with the other, with cause an effect and effect a cause, creates a wholeness which contains the spirit of the moving.

The outer body (muscles-joints-limbs in space-direction-placement) and the inner mind (awareness-attention-perception) are always in touch with each other. With the ever-present structural harmony, the movements shape the developing patterns into significant Form, without which there can be no spirit. The continuous manipulation of the Forms with concentration and consciousness contains and releases a spirit of calm well-being and alert equanimity. To be aware of self and to sense selfless objectivity while in space-time balanced movement is to capture and to experience the Moving Spirit.

From the very first movement of t'ai-chi ch'üan, the mind's presence and the control of a constant continuum urge the spirit to emerge or make the spirit come to life. The body as a physical force, the body as a psychological entity, the mind as the ever-present power, philosophically and practically, all merge harmoniously. This integrated harmony constitutes the spirit and *is* the spirit-centered calm, aware and concentrated.

Even from the very beginning of one's study, at which time form and movement can hardly be understood fully and which certainly cannot be performed correctly, even then, the process of moving in the t'ai-chi ch'üan 'Way', without multiple patterns and balanced dynamics, stirs up a new feeling that is more than physical. It is a 'spirit' inherent in the nature of t'ai-chi ch'üan (and all great art) that touches and envelops even the raw beginner. When comprehension develops in depth and with relative accuracy in rendering the structure, then clearly the quality of the feeling-sensation becomes richer, more subtle and profound.

In essence, t'ai-chi ch'üan is a composite of the art of activity which unites the personality into a totality: the physical self being involved with the mind, the mind stimulating the body, and both together affecting the emotional condition and the spiritual aspect. Functioning physically in the prescribed way with its harmonious complexities and 'united energies', t'ai-chi ch'üan will reveal the nature of the Moving Spirit and the presence of the spirit moving.

Since "that which transforms the form is the spirit" (Binyon, *The Flight of the Dragons*), at the completion of the exercise, with the finishing touch of the final gesture, the feeling-sensation does not disappear. Though the outer activity has ceased, the inner activity goes on. The Moving Spirit penetrates the system for several seconds, and this length of time is increased as one's experience moves one to a higher level of awareness and technique.

Many of us have felt that delicious calm that settles over us when we give ourselves in unselfconscious relaxation to the setting sun and the light of twilight. At that hour, nature creates an almost total stillness, even though the subtle changes in shades of color and shapes of clouds are steadily intermingling.

This feeling is *not* the kind of calm that comes from t'ai-chi ch'üan, where the calm is of our *own* making, and accompanies the Moving Spirit. Whereas we react to and accept the sunset's quieting affect, with t'ai-chi ch'üan we create the quiet through our *willed* activity by recreating harmony. Calm is within us and spreads outwardly, never fading but gradually augmenting with use and self growth.

The calmness of sunset touches us from the outside inward, and although we respond most agreeably to it, it does not have the power to change us from inside out, except temporarily. The sunset's calm has a settling effect, we become *be-calmed*. But t'ai-chi ch'üan produces the opposite result; we acquire an enlivening, a *vital* calm which the Moving Spirit promises to make permanent.

## A Harmony of Change

Embedded in the very nature of t'ai-chi ch'üan is the principle that every aspect of its continually moving process must be made to be harmonious. This principle, the essence of mind-body equilibrium directs the content, organizes the form, and diversifies the motion so that all becomes a harmony of change in balanced proportions.

Just as organic matter is in a state of continual change and motion, so the man-made exercise of t'ai-chi ch'üan is an image of nature's fundamental way. The t'ai-chi ch'üan changes have been made harmonious by men and women's understanding of their own natures and by their optimistic belief in the possibility of continual development on higher planes of self-knowlege.

Such harmony presumes the refined interaction of the physical and mental, the instinctive and the psychological, with the organized and organic principles of the *T'ai Chi*—the philosophical way, and of the *Ch'üan*—the physical way. Harmony is the intrinsic relationship of all the structure's qualities intercontrolled.

Harmony at every part of the moving whole is felt at each "caught" moment of the configurations which balance space, position, energy, weight, and lightness. Harmony is felt at every motion in the forming patterns as each subtly connects with what follows in terms of physiology and in terms of the eight directions for space.

Simultaneous as a chord in music, each separate patterned t'ai-chi ch'üan form is a single chord of action. T'ai-chi ch'üan, as a complete exercise, can be considered a *total* chord in the light of it having attained the integration of meaning and method.

T'ai-chi ch'üan becomes a highly complex synthesis which is the result of harmonious fusion of the multiplicity of changing elements balanced at every stage of the exercise's involved activity.

To be aware of the multiplicity of change does not disturb the mind nor distract the self from being centered to attend to the differentiations. Instead, it develops acute sensibility and the mature ability to perceive the *wholeness* as being more significant than the many-shaded combinations within it. Because all changes are created to move consistently and organically in terms of gravity, the dynamic (yin-yang) use of engergy is harmonious with the ever-progressing process of change.

With mind in control, the physical body is propelled willingly, smoothly, and flowingly from one movement to another without any emotion interfering with or influencing even the most subtle unit.

Nonetheless, rising spontaneously, a "feeling" response appears, clear and definite, which can be described as a sensitive sensing of the harmonious nature of what is being enacted at all times. Agreeable, comforting, calming, with a glow of satisfaction—this is the composite and the pervasive feeling. When body and mind function in unity continually, this initial feeling, this pleasurable reaction, is gradually transformed into a higher state—that of containment, secure and serene.

As a "philosophy" of physical discipline integrating mind-feeling with the nurturing of the internal/external bodily system, t'ai-chi ch'üan unites *all* (changes) into *one* (harmony) and thus succeeds in making 'oneness of all', a harmony of change.

The design for T'ai-chi is the subtle symbol for the balanced philosophy and the physiological processes which comprise t'ai-chi ch'üan. The double wave line centered in a circle epitomizes the grace of flowing space in all the structured action of this exercise-art. The boundary of the circle keeps shape and movement under control within its wholeness. The double turn within it makes an infinity of forms move as if in unlimited and free exchange.

The circle and the wave produce all shades of differentiation in yin-yang interchange. Necessarily related, the dual activity of this dynamic interplay results in balance impeccably adjusted in the ever-changing patterns of this many-faceted composition.

The essence of unity is embodied in the concept of such duality—action-movement and the dynamic changes as wave, and stillness-quiescence as circle.

We weave a circle of containment around us as we follow the continuous circular paths which form t'ai-chi ch'üan structure. Unwittingly, we create a field of energy within us as we experience the rhythmic ebb and flow of the dynamic changes inherent in the nature of the wave.

When we perform with physiological accuracy the motion of wave and circle in their proper proportions, we will be in perfect coordinated balance. The circle is 'an urge to wholeness', and the wave is ceaseless change. The circle, though it may be thought of as a finite circumference, is yet capable of limitless expansion. The wave may seem boundless, but framed as it is by the embracing circle, it does have its spatial limitations.

The interweaving wave patterns have a destination—that of becoming Form. Form is the union of balanced space-time relationships that have momentarily culminated (climaxed) in a completed structure which is felt as total stillness (yin), the yang or motion patterns having gradually transformed themselves into yin structure. Form as an ending, however, does not cease or stop; its completeness, sensed, sets a new beginning into motion. It is as if one had rounded out a circle which, as Form, contains the seed of new action.

Form can be considered to express the contained and calm spirit of circle and motion, the process which materializes the form. The Way of the Wave Action (which is what the T'ai-chi is) is the means by which to advance to the Meaning. This is the heart of the process of t'ai-chi ch'üan.

The Forms (108 in all) are each a unique state of awareness. Each represents a peak experience in the evolving process of self-development which, like the circle, has unbounded possibilities for profound expansion.

"The T'ai-chi is the symbol of the universe"—Professor Joseph Needham

T'ai-chi ch'üan speaks for itself in the exquisite smoothness of its activity, in the quiet flow of its dynamic movement and in the lyricism of its tempo.

Awareness of the paths of moving, concentration on the way of movement, produce a magnetic vibration which makes the lack of sound go unnoticed. Not heard but felt, the inner voice of t'ai-chi ch'üan speaks out, is sensed (though not quite understood) by anyone who comes within the visible field of its activity.

Unprepared as I was for t'ai-chi ch'üan when first I saw it in Peking, I responded to it as if it spoke out to me personally. The unaccompanied movement in structured balances projected a quiescence not only as if 'aural', but also emotional, and I felt a magnetism which seemed to send forth meaning and essence.

T'ai-chi ch'üan needs no outside influence of sound accompaniment to lean on, to interpret, or to speak for it. We can say that it sings out and fills the air with an orchestrated composition which has a resonance that amplifies itself with structured variations of spaced time, phrased themes, and with subtly textured inner/outer harmonies. In "concert", all project a quiet which is distinctly heard.

This quiet speaks to us as does the silent dawn, which is not at all like the deep silence of midnight nor like the stillness of fading twilight. Dawn-quiet is fresh and bright and seems to promise a new awakening.

So t'ai-chi ch'üan resumed each day acquires new clarity, develops depth of insight as to what we can say to ourselves as we "listen" to it.

With the external silence of t'ai-chi ch'üan which helps to make the mind less noisy, with quiet attention and calm spirit, we can hear the inner voice of t'ai-chi ch'üan make its meaning become more and more resoundingly clear. As time goes on and experiences accumulate, t'ai-chi ch'üan and its way of silence vibrate more eloquently.

## Spontaneity: The Look of Ease

Spontaneity in doing t'ai-chi ch'üan comes after long, repeated practice of the entire exercise. When all is ingrained in the system and consciously directed, only then does t'ai-chi ch'üan activity have the effect of being performed with spontaneity—as if with no thought and no mind.

Spontaneity arises not only from the feeling of familiarity and the accomplishment of every detail spatially and physiologically, but also *especially* from deep comprehension of the spirit of the whole.

If one is to appear spontaneous and to experience ease, no awkward movements, no intrinsic forcing, no mechanical rendering of patterns and positions are possible or permissible. No emotional or temperamental moods may color the action. These all would disrupt the inner process of ease—ease which is the ultimate quality leading the way toward spontaneity.

It is commonly thought that a spontaneous art springs from the heart without any thought interference—out of nowhere into the light of day. A sudden decision to behave in a certain way is often termed spontaneous. But the cause for action may have been embedded in the mind for some time, awaiting the propitious moment to be put into external action.

This is *not* the spontaneity of t'ai-chi ch'üan. An analogy to what occurs in t'ai-chi ch'üan, where the effect is spontaneous, when the content and technique have been thoroughly studied, is that of the performing pianist, whose trained fingers glide over the keyboard perfectly with all the expressive nuances seemingly executed without any thought. Only after years of practice, acquiring technical skills and understanding of musical essence, can the pianist produce, without effort, the atmosphere of spontaneity.

The same approach applies to the t'ai-chi ch'üan players. When every aspect has been learned excellently, the entire exercise becomes so much a part of the person that t'ai-chi ch'üan appears to be unstudied. Then it truly has the look, the easy look, of spontaneity—almost as if it were being improvised freely.

Being in complete *control* at all times—which means recognizing and conforming to the principles of the philosophy and structure of the activity—constitutes the essence of spontaneity. For instance, when one is writing and the words move smoothly along the page, the brain and the hand are simultaneously in control. The letter, the word, and the concepts emanate from knowledge, and it is knowledge in any activity that gives control. Therefore the act of writing, flowing unhesitatingly, seems free but is actually controlled by knowledge, with mind centered and aware.

In t'ai-chi ch'üan, one senses a feeling of satisfaction in being in control of oneself in relation to the exercise and in being in control of the exercise in terms of one's self. One feels free and at ease in experiencing the exercise as being under one's control.

Such freedom is framed by knowledge—being sure of all apsects of t'ai-chi ch'üan with mind in control. The appearance is that of spontaneity, the inner feeling is that of freedom, secure and easy.

Because of the innate harmony of all elements in the structure of t'ai-chi ch'üan, this exercise cannot but produce an organically organized reaction— that of being in total balance. With the development of increasing knowledge and control, both freedom and spontaneity ensue progressively. The look of ease, the air of spontaneity will arise inevitably, and t'ai-chi ch'üan, to quote grand master Ma Yüeh-liang in Shanghai, will become "second nature."

At the completion of t'ai-chi ch'üan, having made "a full circle round" with awareness, a singular sense of harmony is experienced.

Spatially and physically the patterned forms have traveled in many directions, touching at different times all points of the compass in a 360° circle. This fact, in itself, is not the only reason for the awakened feeling of fulfillment. It is due to the total composition: to the curvilinear nature of the continuous movement; to the minutely harmonious relationship of 'all' that is taking place; to the presence of the mind in 'amity' with body-action.

The "full-circle" is physically and psychologically the expression of body-mind-space-time-structured-harmony, all coordinated to a fraction of a minute. The moment of the "ending" is a stay of action alerting one to the stillness within—a feeling akin to what is felt at the beginning but with a difference. The ending stillness contains the essence of containment on a very deep level. The beginning stillness is mentally induced; the ending stillness having grown intrinsically in the process of experiencing the structure as a whole, pervades the entire being: the feeling, body and mind.

The action of t'ai-chi ch'üan having traversed a large world of space and shape, finally arrives at the position (bodily and spatially) in which the exercise began. Though externally similar as are the body stances at the beginning and the ending, the spirit *however* at the ending is very different— obviously—since the practitioner has moved through a world of harmonious changes and is hardly the *same* as when he or she began.

What is extremely interesting is the developing keenness of consciousness as one moves through the ever-changing harmonies of the multiple forms.

At the close, all complexities of action disappear to become a simple unit of movement, as was the original stance.

Physically and mentally, the two stances are not the same: the *start* opens to awaken the yin and yang dynamic; the *finish* is "neutral", containing no feeling of differentiation in the torso or legs. All is light (yet non-moving), as if magically suspended.

Whereas the attention at the start is poised for action, the mind at the end is centered in stillness.

At every stage of "advancement" in t'ai-chi ch'üan a more profound element is generated, which makes the ending more gratifying and elated.

Whatever the final sensation is, a comfortable calmness lingers on intrinsically for a long time after moving away from t'ai-chi ch'üan's final moment.

When t'ai-chi ch'üan is resumed on another day, it is always on a more elevated level of awareness. Each repetition advances to yet another height, to reveal deeper and richer insight.

Photographs in the many Chinese magazines I have seen show groups of elderly men in t'ai-chi ch'üan positions, seemingly moving in unison. Does this make it an old person's exercise, or does it imply that it is an exercise which people, only when older, should learn? Neither is true. T'ai-chi ch'üan is an exercise to get older *with*.

By practicing t'ai-chi ch'üan for years and years, one will arrive at a good old age with comfort and health. Therefore, t'ai-chi ch'üan is a young person's exercise, and my reasoning is simple. It must be learned and studied when one is younger, and it must be practiced and perfected day after day, year after year, in order to reach a ripe old age with stamina and mental agility. Since t'ai-chi ch'üan is known as an exercise aiming toward longevity, it must necessarily be started a long time before the great age arrives.

From my teaching experience, I have found that older people (in the United States) who have not exercised when younger have great difficulty in coordinating not only mind with body but also hands and feet. Even if the older person lacks *physical* strength, it does not hamper learning. It is the inability of the mind to be attentive and the body to coordinate with it—as well as the lack of willpower to persist—which are the basic reasons for the older person's difficulties in studying.

Since it is the ever-changing variety of forms and patterns which are designed to produce balanced health, fine circulation, and pliable muscles and joints, it can be seen how important it is to function with *that* variety so uniquely contained in t'ai-chi ch'üan. Therefore, a modicum of the ability to concentrate and coordinate must be present from the very beginning of study. The intricate diversity led by the mind stimulates it to become more keenly perceptive and ever present. It is the subtle variety which keeps the dynamics of changing energies in moving balance and which brings new and fresh life to the entire system.

It stands to reason, then, that people must start to learn when they are young enough—at that time when they are able to press the mind into attention and to develop the memory more easily, to make the body act in a multitude of ways physiologically, and especially to have the will to persevere with the thought being not on *old* or *any* age, but on physical, emotional, and mental self-development.

How young is young? The twenties are not too young, and certainly the forties and fifties are never too late. But, I do believe that the teens are much too young, too early in life experience to be objective and to understand the concept of mental and emotional equilibrium. The teens are the time for exercising with tensed strength, extrinsically, with clearly felt and vigorous physicality. T'ai-chi ch'üan requires another kind of mind and muscle intelligence. It demands acute attention, intrinsic and quiet control, and the appreciation and awareness of human potentialities.

People over twenty can give themselves to a new experience willingly and can begin to detect the refinements of a more subtle kind on a more philosophical plane.

Learning at the right time, at a good mental age, one can move through the decades staying young as one's years accumulate. With its structural and philosophical harmony, t'ai-chi ch'üan can be considered to be a mature exercise at any age. It is an exercise which all people, as they get older, can continue to do with ease. T'ai-chi ch'üan can be designated as "old" if the t'ai-chi ch'üan player has lived a long time—long enough to have become wiser while maintaining an active, healthy body and a clear, agile mind. T'ai-chi ch'üan is an exercise for men and women of any age to stay young with.

## The Student is Forever

Is it a discouraging or an optimistic thought that the student is forever? It would be depressing if the student remained forever on the same level of meager knowledge or even on an advanced one, or did not see the possibility for further growth or perceive that there was more to know. When the goals are recognized as profound and when the technique, though complex, is enticing as well, the idea that the learning is forever is invigorating.

To know is to want to know more, which indicates that there is more to know, an ever-satisfying progress. However, it would be frustrating to contemplate "forever" as a perpetual state if each "knowing" point were not in itself an agreeable whole, a completeness that radiates quiet pleasure and which leads to another more searching experience. This is the promise of t'ai-chi ch'üan at all moments.

Just as artists always feel themselves to be on the road to greater creativity, just as inventors move ahead after fulfilling one idea which in turn may be the seed of another, so the student (at any level) is perpetually moving ahead in depth, in physical stamina, in mental discernment of the objective exercise, and in the more subtle awareness of self and especially of some unique, harmonious experience within.

To repeat t'ai-chi ch'üan as *only* a physical exercise is impossible. Impossible because the mental and physical are intrinsically united in this exercise. All the elements coexist and are revealed at the very same moment of action. And these seep into the system of even the most ignorant, eventually to reach conscious levels of awareness. To do is to know and to know is to do more and more with ever-increasing ease and sensitivity.

But being a student does not always imply the presence of a teacher-in-command. Being able to be a student by oneself, of and for oneself, proves the vital and constant growth in thinking, feeling, and doing of a more highly developed person.

No matter how great the master-teacher is (or was), the furthering of knowledge and experience becomes the *matter* for self-penetration and illumination. Only from such self-progress can comprehension arise which further lights up the entire subject of t'ai-chi ch'üan as a balance of harmonious change. The perception of the material and the immaterial elements of t'ai-chi ch'üan continues to develop in the 'forever student' under his or her own masterful eye and mind.

And when the student becomes a master on other levels of comprehension, he or she is, nevertheless, a student experiencing, perceiving, developing forever.

## CHAPTER 11

*Metaphorically and symbolically, all quotations included are pertinent to the philosophy, technique and structure of t'ai-chi ch'üan, in spirit, action, study, practice and experience.*

*The I-Ching quotations are culled from the* Book of Changes, *the Richard Wilhelm translation, rendered into English by Cary F. Baynes, Bollingen Series XIX, Pantheon Books, 1950. (The numbers refer to the pages in the hard-cover version.) All other quotations come from a wide range of sources, as indicated by author and book.*

**Calmness-Perseverance-Concentration**

*From The I-Ching*

He who stays calm will succeed in making things go well in the end. *(26)*

It is only through *gentleness* that this can have a successful outcome. *(42)*

To carry out our purpose we need firm determination within and gentleness and adaptability in external relationships. *(42)*

True quiet means keeping still when the time has come to keep still, and going forward when the time has come to go forward. *(214)*

If the movement of the spinal nerves is brought to a standstill, the ego, with its restlessness disappears, as it were. When a man has become *calm*, he may turn to the outside world. *(215)*

. . . calmness must develop naturally out of a state of inner composure *(216)*.

True joy rests on firmness and strength within, manifesting itself outwardly as yielding and gentle. *(238)*

. . . within its tranquility, which guards against precipitous actions, and without its penetration, which makes development and progress possible. *(218)*

. . . shows tranquil beauty—*clarity* within, quiet without. *(97)*

If one is serious and composed he can acquire the *clarity* of mind needed for coming to terms with the innumerable impressions that pour in. *(128)*

It is precisely at the beginning that serious *concentration* is important, because the beginning holds the seeds of all that is to follow. *(128)*

. . . man's thoughts should restrict themselves to the immediate situation. *(215)*

We must know how to enjoy the moment without being deflected from the goal, for perseverance is needed to remain victorious. *(27)*

Only this combination of inner strength and outer reserve enables one to take on responsibility . . . *(23)*

If fellowship is to lead to order there must be *order* within diversity. *(59)*

Everything proceeds as if on its own accord, and this can all too easily tempt us to relax and let things take their course without troubling over details. *(261)*

### Philosophy-Structure

In order to find one's place in the infinity of being, one must be able both to separate and to unite. *(17)*

. . . there is also created the idea of duration both in and beyond time, a movement that never stops or slackens, just as one day follows another in an unending course. *(5)*

The movement is cyclic, and the course complete itself. . . . Everything comes of itself at the appointed time. *(104)*

All movements are accomplished in six stages, and the seventh brings return. *(104)*

All that is visible must grow beyond itself, extend into the realm of the invisible. *(206)*

Duration is a state when movement is not worn down by hindrances. It is not a state of rest, for mere standstill is regression. Duration is rather the self-contained and therefore self-renewing movement of an organized, firmly integrated whole, taking place in accordance with immutable laws and beginning anew at every ending. *(135-136)*

. . . every end contains a new beginning. Thus it gives hope to men. *(269)*

. . . unswerving inner purpose brings good fortune in the end. An obstruction that lasts only for a time is useful for self-development. *(162)*

. . . rest is merely a state of polarity that always posits movement as its complement. *(214)*

Because he sees with great clarity causes and effects, he completes the six steps at the right time . . . The six steps are the six different positions of the hexagram . . . each step attained forwith becomes a preparation for the next . . . the means of making actual what is potential. (T'ai-chi ch'üan in the long Wu style has six "series" which are six levels of evolutionary development). *(3)*

. . . based on the polarity of positive and negative principles. *(4)*

Of great importance, furthermore, is the law of movement along the line of least resistance . . . *(70)*

The inviolability of natural laws . . . rests on this principle of movement along the line of least resistance. These laws are not forces external to things but represent the harmony of movement immanent in them. *(71)*

Movement . . . must be strengthened by rest, so that it will not be dissipated by being used prematurely. *(104-105)*

If a leg is suddenly stopped while the whole body is in vigorous motion, the continuing body movement will make one fall. *(216)*

What is not sought in the right way is not found. *(137)*

Form no longer conceals content but brings out its values in full. Perfect grace consists not in exterior ornamentation of the substance, but in the simple fitness of the form. *(99)*

Pleasure shared is pleasure doubled. *(44)*

There are people who live in a state of perpetual hurry without ever attaining inner composure. Restlessness not only prevents all thoroughness but actually becomes a danger . . . *(138)*

### Teaching-Learning

. . . a man who is good at his work is content to behave simply. He wishes to make progress in order to accomplish something. When he attains his goal, he does something worthwhile and all is well. *(47)*

. . . discipline should not degenerate into drill. Continuous drill has a humiliating effect and cripples a man's powers. *(22)*

An inexperienced person who seeks instruction in a childlike and unassuming way is on the right path, for the man devoid of arrogance who subordinates himself to his teacher will certainly be helped. *(23)*

. . . in teaching others everything depends on consistency for it is only through repetition that a pupil makes the material his own. *(123)*

No situation can become favorable until one is able to adapt to it and does not wear himself out with mistaken resistance. *(76)*

The very gradualness of the development makes it necessary to have perseverance, for perseverance alone prevents slow progress from dwindling to nothing. *(219)*

The tree . . . does not shoot up like a swamp plant; its growth proceeds gradually. Thus also the work of influencing people can only be gradual. No sudden influence of awakening of lasting effect. Progress must be made gradual . . . *(219)*

He who demands too much at once is acting precipitously, and because he attempts too much, he ends by succeeding in nothing. *(137)*

Knowledge should be a refreshing and vitalizing force. It becomes so only through stimulating intercourse with congenial friends with whom one holds discussion. . . . In this way learning becomes many-sided and takes on a cheerful lightness, whereas there is always something ponderous and one sided about the learning of the self-taught. *(239)*

. . . Finally where the moods of his own heart are concerned, he should never ignore the possibility of inhibition, for this is the basis for human freedom. *(133)*

*From Other Sources*

It is the property of intelligence to perceive things in germination.

Lao Tzu

Each race contributes something essential to the world's civilization in the course of its own self-expression and self-realization.

Ananda Coomaraswamy
*The Dance of Siva*

There is a whole gamut of latent faculties and invisible forces which considerably surpass the possibilities of our surface beings . . . one has to have the passage clear between the outer mind and the inner being.

Sri Aurobindo
*The Adventure of Consciousness*

To remember oneself is to be quiet. . . . One must have patience to weave a long life.

Paul Valery

I am constantly anxious lest the meaning should not match the object of attention, lest the artistic form should not reach the level of the meaning.

Lu Chi *The Art of Letters*
as translated by E. R. Hughes

Although painting is representation of form, it is dominated by idea . . . as the idea is in the form, it cannot be expressed if the form is neglected. When the form is grasped, it will fill the idea completely; but when the form is lost, how can there be either form or idea?

Wang Li in *The Chinese on the
Art of Painting* by Osvald Siren

To understand the significance of a thing, one must become the thing, harmonize one's consciousness with it and reach the mental attitude which brings knowledge without intellectual deliberation.

Osvald Siren
*The Chinese on the Art of Painting*

All science would be superfluous if the appearance of things coincided directly with their essence.

Karl Marx

The first value of self-knowledge is its usefulness, even necessity, in one's self-correction of the truthfulness of one's experience. . ... The immediate intrinsic value of one's experience depends in part on how much its primitive deep levels can be registered on the high levels of consciousness.

Robert C. Neville
*Soldier, Sage, Saint*

Understanding is the essence obtained from information intentionally learned and from all kinds of experiences personally experienced.

G. I. Gurdieff
*Meetings with Remarkable Men*

The only 'enough' that's enough is to know what is enough.

William McNaughton
*The Taoist Vision*

A cat's energy is subdued into an exquisite moderation. Other animals employ what strength they happen to possess without reference to the smallness of the occasion, but a cat uses only the necessary force.

Philip G. Hammerton

Resources of the spirit are like savings—they must be accumulated before they are needed.

Martin Ten Hoor
*Essay Today*

*Hsu* is not non-existence; it is contained because this emptiness has an essence (soul) connected with the Superbeing (*Shen*) or personality, which connects our bodies 'being.' When '*Shen*' or personality is filled there is agility and freshness, self control and body ease.

Wu Chien-Ch'üan and Ma Yueh-Liang
*Tai-Chi Ch'üan (1935)*

Our striving must be to press back from the periphery towards the centre, from movement to quiescence, from multiplicity to unity, from knowledge to wisdom.

Hans-Ulreich Rieker
*Beggar Among the Dead*

*Shih* means event or Form: "That which is solved by changes is *Shih*" (I-Ching). Form, or event, is more than its static condition. The ever changing event is what is called *Shih*. It is *particularly* in action.

Chang Chung-Yuan
*Creativity and Taoism*

Various postures strictly and intelligently designed to provide body tone, good glandular performance supply serenity to mind.

Plato

Our bodies are gardens wherein our minds are the master.

Shakespeare
*Othello*

In order to apply energy to the body with utmost effect, we must discover a certain related order; when found a power comes into play which far surpasses in effect the application of pure brute strength and muscular effort.

Lawrence Binyon

The Great Balance has no personal power. And its myriad veins interlace of themselves.

T'ao Ch'ien (Poet)
William Archer, translator

Yin and Yang, spirit and matter, the passive and the active are all inexhaustible, indestructible, and equal. All phenomena and effects, visible and invisible are produced by their ceaseless motion and interplay: The Great Balance.

William Archer,
editor, translator, annotator
of T'ao Ch'ien's Poems

T'ai-chi ch'üan is not pure *Tao* which eliminates distinctions. It is relative Tao which recognizes distinctions—scale, proportion, size, relativity. T'ai-chi ch'üan finds the maximum equilibrium.

Chou Hsiang-Kung (Hong Kong)
*The Orient Magazine*

The philosophic and practical goals (consciousness) are given forms which in return gives the idea, which idea is hidden if one is not ready to receive it. . . . Tao is Great Mind

Paul Goulart
*The Monastery of Jade Mountain*

Tao is a cosmic process of both man and nature: interaction of two opposite principles which come from yin and yang, the primordial mixture of matter and energy, in the form of a fluid in gyratory motion.

S. F. Mason
*Main Currents of Scientific Thought*

Eternal rightness restores the mystery to the ordinary.

In t'ai-chi ch'üan you will find semblance of an eagle flying, fish in the deep sea, full of life and vitality. . . . Mysterious is the essence of t'ai-chi ch'üan... It is a game fit for the immortals.

Ch'en Ch'ang Hsing
*Chen's T'ai-Chi Ch'üan: Theory and Illustration*

Even before starting the physical exercise, the state of mind is sufficient to affect the chemistry of blood circulation, vitality and metabolism.

Dr. Ch'u Mien Yu
*T'ai-Chi Ch'üan: Its Exercise and Application*

The mind is always working with three manifestations or energies: matter, being the initial force; *mobility-movement*, creating form and rhythm, and harmony, the composite of spirit.

Murray Gitlin
*Body and Mind and Their Possibilities*

Special honor is paid to the Spirit of the Polar Star identified with T'ai-Chi (the great Limit and Absolute) because it never changes its position with relation to the rest of the universe.

Juliet Bredon
*The Moon Year 1927*
Kelly and Walsh

I am as constant as the Northern Star
  Of whose true-fixed and resting quality
  There is no fellow in the firmament.

Shakespeare<br>Julius Caesar

If you are not patient with little things you will bring great plans to naught.
Chinese Proverb

The perfect man can transcend the limits and yet not withdraw from the world. . . . Those who would benefit mankind from deep forests of lofty mountains are simply unequal to the strain upon their higher natures!
Chuang Tzu

Those move easiest who learn to dance
  From art and not by chance.

Alexander Pope

Intelligence is the ability to undertake activities that are characterized by 1. difficulty, 2. complexity, 3. abstractness, 4. economy, 5. adaptiveness, 6. social value, 7. the emergence of originals, and to maintain such activities under conditions that demand a concentration of energy and a resistance to emotional forces.
Dr. George Stoddard<br>The Meaning of Intelligence<br>quoted by Anthony Smith in The Body

Gladly would he learn; gladly would he teach.
G. Chaucer

Knowledge originates with direct experience. . . .perseverance raises level of consciousness and thus gain understanding and happiness. . . .Combination of opposites—unity of will and personal ease of mind.
Mao Tzu-Tung

A heart at ease flies in no extremes—'tis ever in the center.
Lawrence Sterne<br>Sentimental Journey

. . .To resolve into a unity greater complexities, is to experience greater satisfaction.
Aurobindo<br>The Future Evolution of Men

Conscious evolution is nothing but the process of inner creativity strangely similar to the growth of a seed.

Lizelle Reymond
*To Live Within*

The Chinese were able to achieve the delicate balance between the physical, mental and spiritual which brings to individuals the maximum of contentment and happiness.

Verne Dyson
*The Yellow Springs*

. . .one of the first wrong assumptions is: that we do not realize that we have to learn that control is a question of knowledge and skill.

Ouspensky
*The Forth Way*

My body is there to hold my brain.

T. Edison

Take account of changed conditions and suit its measures to the age.

Chuang-Tzu

The mind is the lord of man's body. Man is heaven, earth is its minister.

Chinese proverb

Man manifests his spirit by acting on concrete situations which confront him. . . .Conduct of alchemy is in one's heart.

*The Philosophy of Wang Yang-Ming*
Translated by F.G. Henke

Only the master can find satisfaction in the mind and only then when it is at one with the heart.

Hans-Ulrich Rieker
*Beggar Among the Dead*

The truer the movement and the greater its content, the slower the swing of the universal pendulum.

Laurence van der Post

Movement and Being:
*A Prose Poem on the Ancient Chinese Art T'ai-Chi Ch'üan*

**1. THIS IS THE WAY IT IS**
Soft and smooth, slow in time, heedful
Of man's needs and nature's laws,
An art-in-movement T'ai-Chi Ch'üan
Creates a being integrated
With itself,—an active, thinking,
Feeling man; engenders heart-mind
Ease; develops wondrous stamina
Beyond the age of ordinary
Retrogression and decay.

The exercise evolves, centered, quiet,
With mind-awareness animating
All the body's actions—from patterns
Simple and symmetrical to complex
Weaving of relationships in
Intricate variety. Forms arise,
Taking shape with myriad subtleties
Each instant balanced and secure—
　　A unity of multiplicities.

**2. THE GREAT BALANCE**
The body moves itself around in
Space, in many figured forms, young in
Legs, mature in mind, the spirit bright.
A harmony in structure and in
Quality. The balances of Yin
And Yang, like shadow and its light
Are poised; though opposite, are friendly.
And compatible, both constantly in
Motion, interchanging equally.

Gathering and separating.
In-out-low-high, solid-void, concrete
And intangible, stillness and
Activity, airiness and weightedness
Molding all in varying degrees
Of intensities; the seeds of one
Come to a fruitful finish which
Itself becomes a new beginning
　　Endlessly unending.

**3. SOFT-INTRINSIC ENERGY**
Feet firmly in control of gravity,
Head and arms float and soar, all
Weightless as in stratosphere.
In supple action joints are joined
Like wave to wavelet on a quiet sea.
Muscles move in flexion and release
As easily as flower-petals
Open-close for light and night
Yielding to necessity.

Ease produced from strength unseen
So gliding ducks seem effortless
Their forceful motion hidden
From the surface of the water;
Outer calm and inner power
Lightness and stability
Agility and energy
Co-exist in T'ai-Chi Ch'üan
　　A magical duality.

## 4. FORM AND SUBSTANCE

The outer form distils in outer air
A radiating calm; it circulates
The inner air, the Ch'i, to inner
Places "subtle as a poet's turn."
Form touches outer air at eight points
Of the compass; these "eight" with "five"
Directions, forward-backward, left-right-
Center, identify themselves with
Diverse universal elements.

Mountain-marsh
Heaven-earth, water-fire
Wood and metal, earth (as matter)
Summer-winter
Spring and autumn,
A positive composite
Greater than the self
Thus making self
    A greater possibility.

## 5. STILLNESS AND ACTIVITY

Lightly, evenly and in balance,
With liquid continuity, patterns
Pass from one part of the body
To the other, each growing out of
That which went before. The subtle
Sequence of this chain unfolds
Invisibly as does the change
From day to dusk to dark to light,
Smooth as a ring of cloudless sky.

The atmosphere of peaceful quiet
Pervades the Being and the Movement
At each measured moment—
The right gesture
At the right time
In the right place
For the right reason, all together
Simultaneous and synchronized
    Is the art of grace refined.

## 6. ORGANIC CHANGE

Action uncoils, interlacing
Shape to Form, reshaping time and space,
Flowing-rolling on with force inside—
Gentleness outside, like water spreading
Down a shallow slope persuasively,
Filling crevices with nonchalance,
Designing forms and changing course
According to the nature
Of the changing situation.

Waving-curving, arcing-circling,
Ebbing-flowing, immense or small,
From obvious to delicate,
The T'ai-Chi Way of Movement
Fits the Forms of Being
In every subtle turn and minute spot,
Dynamics interplaying
Alternating with the nature
    Of the changes changing.

## 7. MIND-ATTENTION

As the eye when focussed on a point
Sees it and all the space around
Completely in a circle, so the mind
When centered, is the eye of consciousness
Controlling, omnipresent and aware;
Like a magnet-beam, the master, mind,
Manipulates with spontaneity
The multi-faceted diversities
Of shape and form and space and time.

Thought and process interwoven
Motion moving without stopping
Create the moment harmonized,
Concentration-integration,
One with all and all at once,
Like a shadow's contact with its source,
Awareness of one's Being, being
Constant with one's self in one embrace
  Is triumph of the power of mind and will.

## 8. MIND-HEART INTENTION

Infinite in its effect is change
Of matter due to T'ai-Chi action;
No trace of tension shows in energy,
Dynamic balance conquers strain and stress,
Vitality is free from nervousness
And strength evolves with pliancy.
Attention centered on the action
Kindles patience, poise, tranquility
And equilibrium in continuum.

Satisfaction with oneself
Is not enough; the centered being
Sensitized, includes a circle
Larger than the self; the silent sounds
Of T'ai-Chi Ch'üan reverberate
With essence of responsibility
To conduct, work and daily life;
To do as well as think and be,
  Is an intrinsic necessity.

## 9. "AND DAILY IT IS NEW"

T'ai-Chi Ch'üan is *lived* not "played at"
In the process of each doing,
Unifying meaning-movment,
Logic-symbol, structure-substance,
Fact and image interactions,
Real and magic interweavings,
Dynamic and organic; body ease
With easy breath and quiet heart, comes
From cultivation of the natural.

Creating calm, longevity,
Keener insight and awareness
To society and self, T'ai-Chi Ch'üan
Completes a circle (cycle), expressed
In matter (form) and motion (breath),
With time not counting time (as space)
Returning to the point where it began,
With consciousness enlivened,
  Finding, in the end, a new beginning.

# Explanation of Foot-Chart

1. The area-space to be covered in the exercise is within a rectangle, 7 by 14 feet—the 'foot' length being in proportion to the person's foot (see pg. 168)

2. Many separate rectangles are used in order to see and follow the sequence of foot placements more clearly.

3. Each rectangle is divided into two areas by an East-West 'axis' line. The space to the South of it is two squares wide; to the North of it (to the front lined demarcation) is five squared feet. The fourteen horizontal squares are so numbered; the vertical ones are delineated as being B' A'/ A B C D E.

4. The right foot-print is light; the left is darkened. The right-left foot positions are connected in a V shape, by dashed lines pointing to a *Figure* and/or *Form* number as illustrated in this book. The last of the right-left foot positions (for each rectangle) is carried over to the following rectangle and is distinguished—from what is to continue—by being marked with *'Striped'* lines.

5. In each rectangle there are two 'dots' placed at the 4th space inward from the East and at the A' vertical space. These dots symbolize the toes of the feet placed at that point of the axis line. This place is significant since it marks both the starting and the finishing foot-stance placement. The dots have been placed in each rectangle to facilitate the organization of the floor patterns since direction and proper placement are essential to the structural totality and essence of this composite exercise.

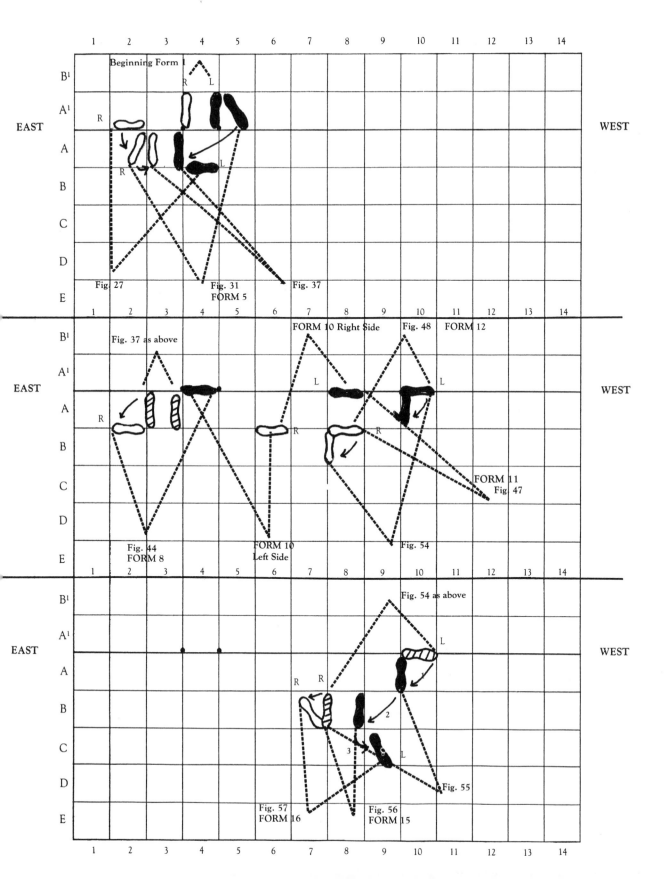

SERIES I-Beginning

Beginning Form 1

Fig. 27    Fig. 31    Fig. 37
FORM 5

Fig. 37 as above

FORM 10 Right Side    Fig. 48    FORM 12

FORM 11
Fig. 47

Fig. 44    FORM 10    Fig. 54
FORM 8    Left Side

Fig. 54 as above

Fig. 55

Fig. 57    Fig. 56
FORM 16    FORM 15

EAST    WEST

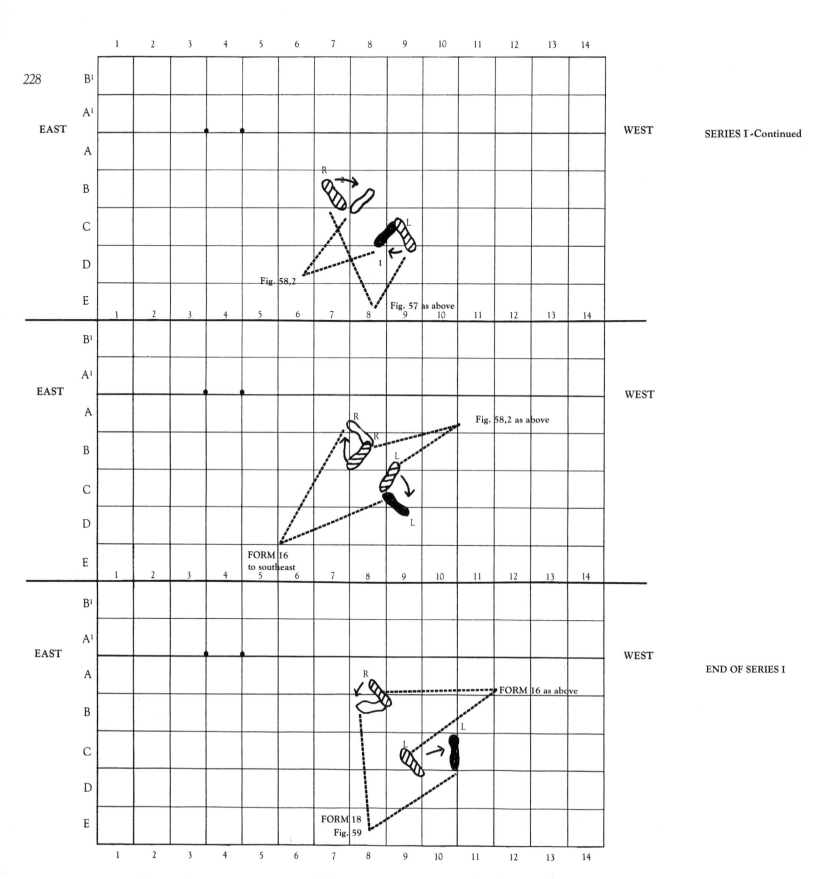

228

EAST — WEST — SERIES I -Continued

R
2
Fig. 58,2
L
1
Fig. 57 as above

EAST — WEST

R
R
Fig. 58,2 as above
L
L
FORM 16
to southeast

EAST — WEST — END OF SERIES I

R
FORM 16 as above
L
L
FORM 18
Fig. 59

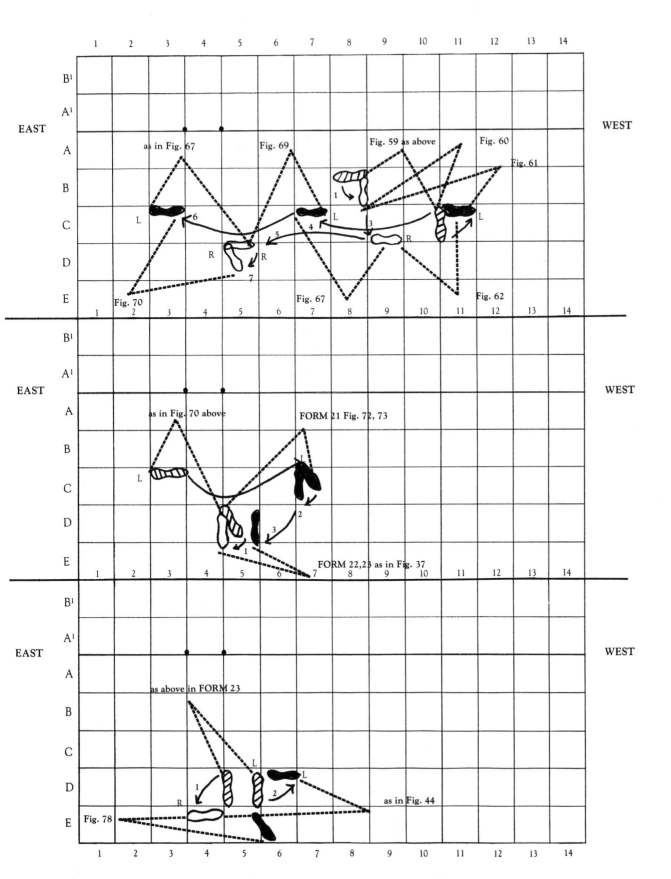

SERIES II-Beginning

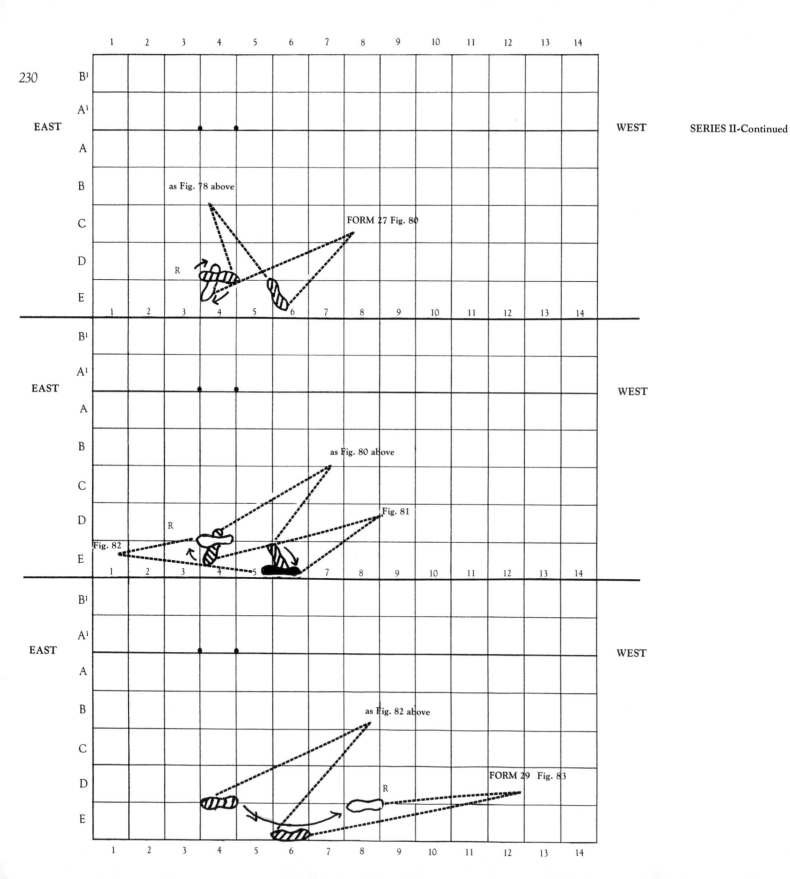

as Fig. 78 above

FORM 27 Fig. 80

R

as Fig. 80 above

Fig. 82

R

Fig. 81

as Fig. 82 above

FORM 29  Fig. 83

R

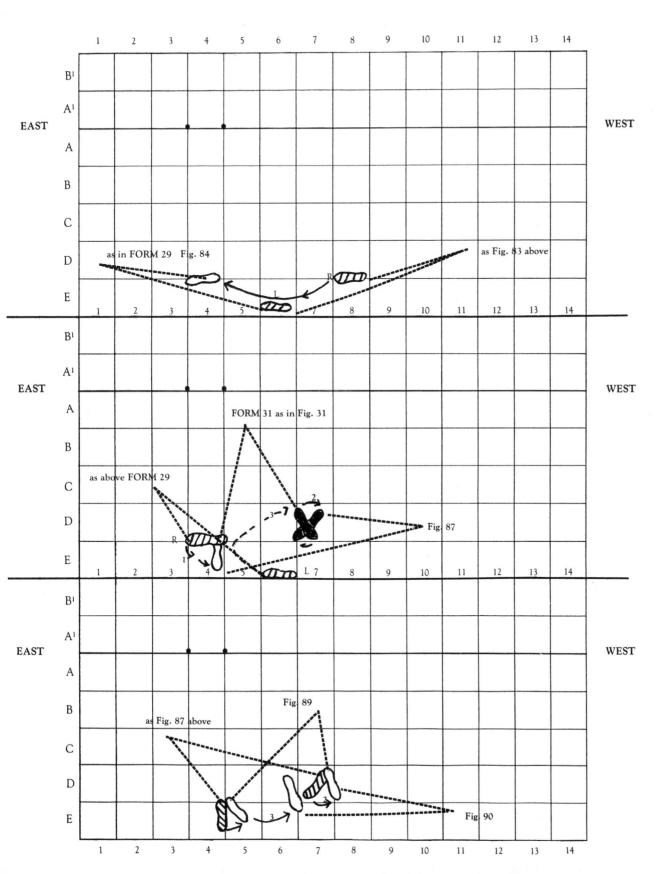

as in FORM 29  Fig. 84

as Fig. 83 above

FORM 31 as in Fig. 31

as above FORM 29

Fig. 87

as Fig. 87 above

Fig. 89

Fig. 90

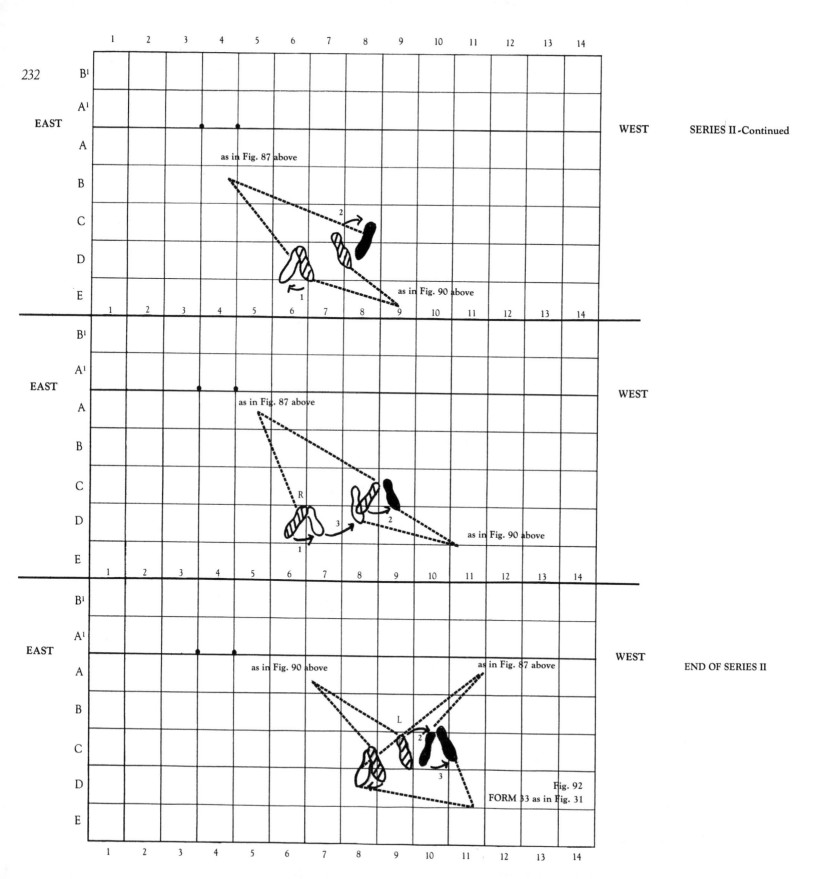

232

EAST · WEST · SERIES II-Continued

as in Fig. 87 above

2

as in Fig. 90 above

1

EAST · WEST

as in Fig. 87 above

R

3

2

1

as in Fig. 90 above

EAST · WEST · END OF SERIES II

as in Fig. 90 above

as in Fig. 87 above

L

2

3

Fig. 92
FORM 33 as in Fig. 31

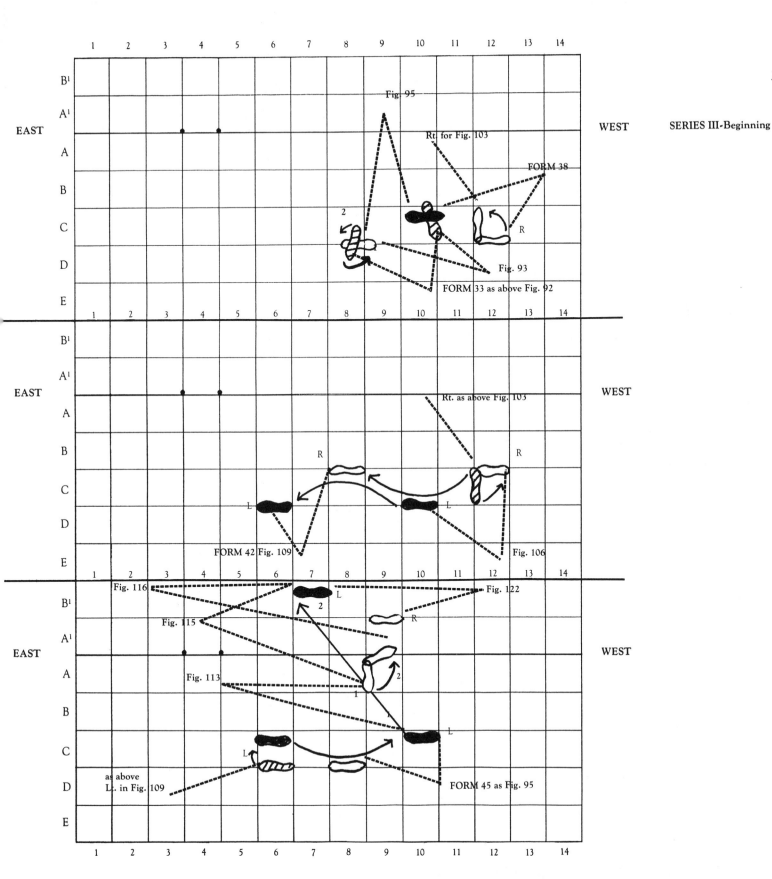

SERIES III-Beginning

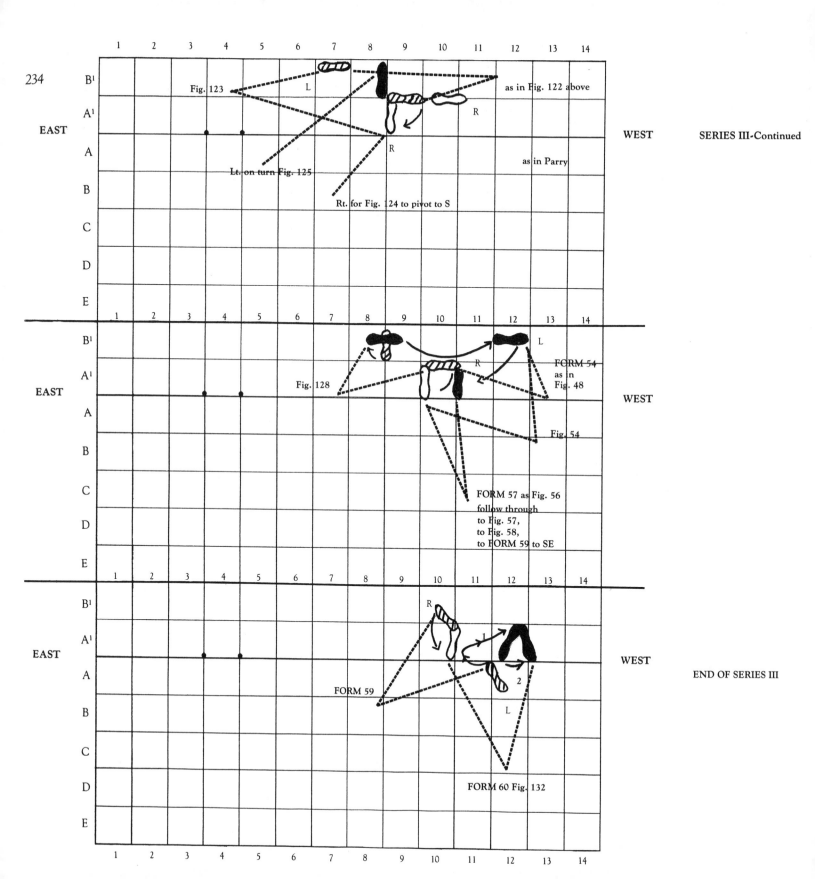

234

EAST

B¹

A¹

Fig. 123

L

as in Fig. 122 above

R

A

R

as in Parry

Lt. on turn Fig. 125

B

Rt. for Fig. 124 to pivot to S

C

D

E

WEST

SERIES III-Continued

EAST

B¹

L

Fig. 128

R

FORM 54
as in
Fig. 48

A¹

A

Fig. 54

B

C

FORM 57 as Fig. 56
follow through
to Fig. 57,
to Fig. 58,
to FORM 59 to SE

D

E

WEST

EAST

B¹

R

1

A¹

2

A

FORM 59

L

B

C

D

FORM 60 Fig. 132

E

WEST

END OF SERIES III

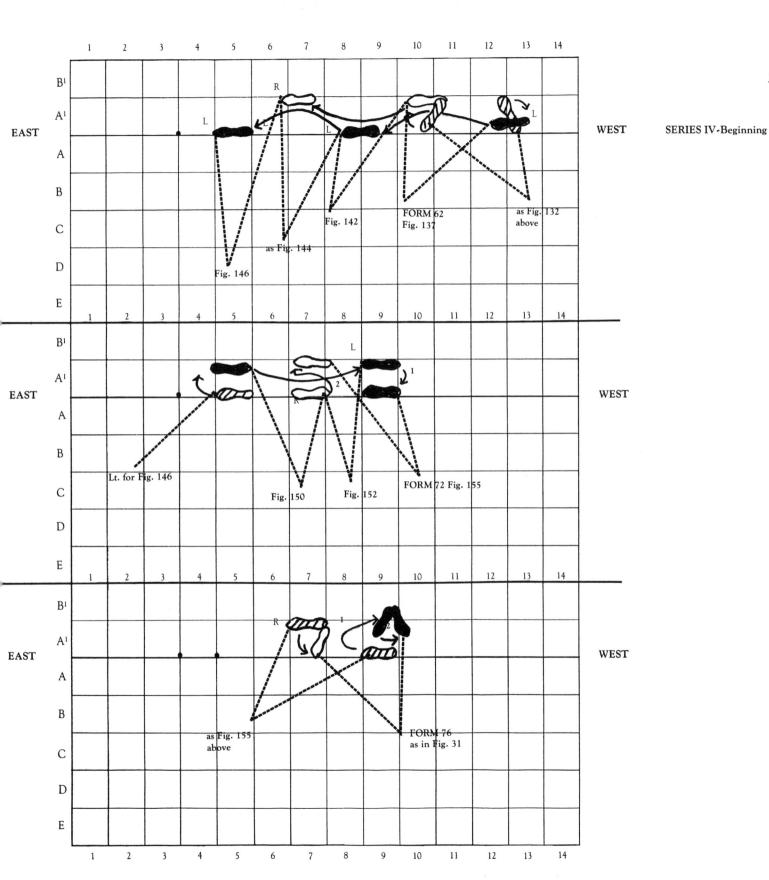

SERIES IV-Beginning

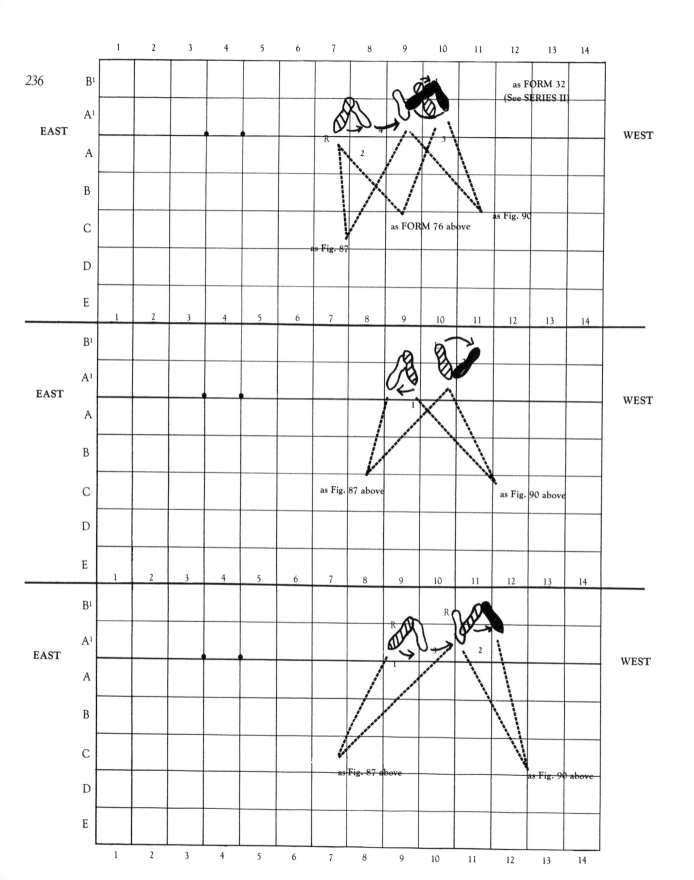

236

EAST

WEST

SERIES IV-Continued

as FORM 32
(See SERIES II)

R

2

4

3

as Fig. 90

as FORM 76 above

as Fig. 87

EAST

WEST

1

as Fig. 87 above

as Fig. 90 above

EAST

WEST

R

R

1

3

2

as Fig. 87 above

as Fig. 90 above

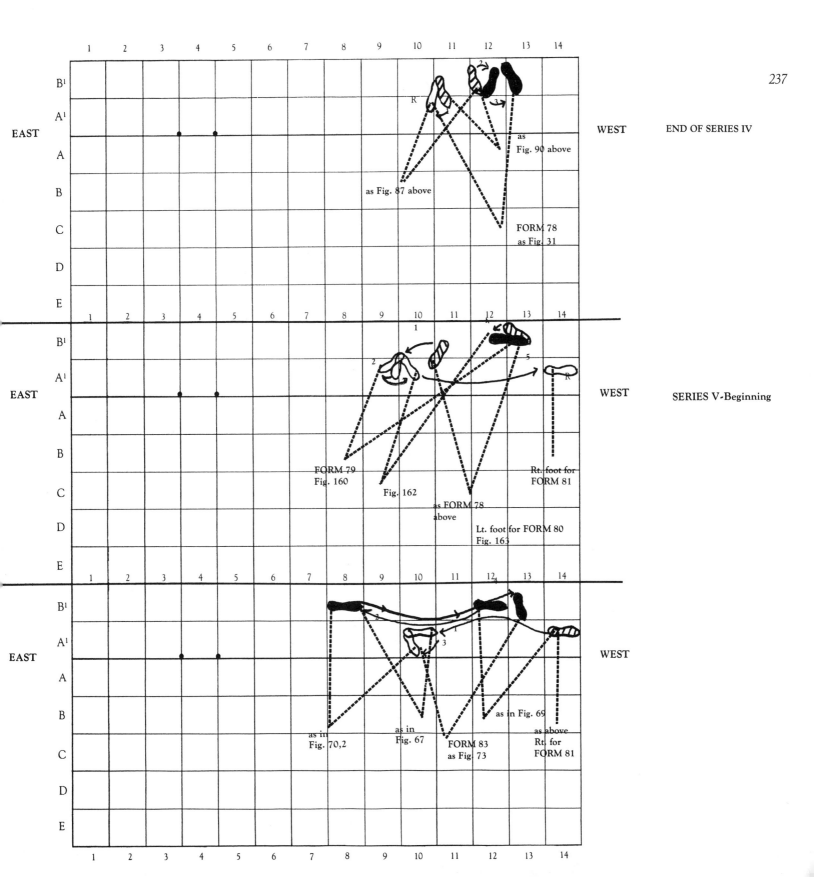

**EAST**      **WEST**      END OF SERIES IV

as
Fig. 90 above

as Fig. 87 above

FORM 78
as Fig. 31

**EAST**      **WEST**      SERIES V-Beginning

FORM 79
Fig. 160

Fig. 162

Rt. foot for
FORM 81

as FORM 78
above

Lt. foot for FORM 80
Fig. 163

**EAST**      **WEST**

as in
Fig. 70,2

as in
Fig. 67

FORM 83
as Fig. 73

as in Fig. 69

as above
Rt. for
FORM 81

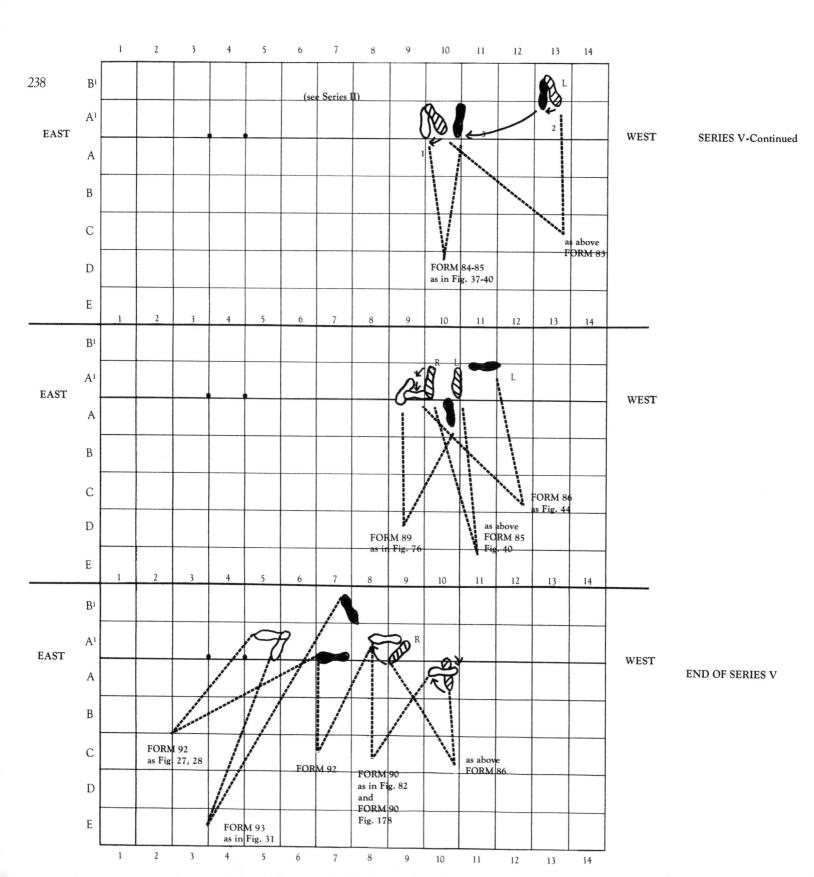

238

EAST     WEST     **SERIES V-Continued**

(see Series II)

FORM 84-85
as in Fig. 37-40

as above
FORM 83

EAST     WEST

FORM 86
as Fig. 44

FORM 89
as in Fig. 76

as above
FORM 85
Fig. 40

EAST     WEST     **END OF SERIES V**

FORM 92
as Fig. 27, 28

FORM 92

FORM 90
as in Fig. 82
and
FORM 90
Fig. 178

as above
FORM 86

FORM 93
as in Fig. 31

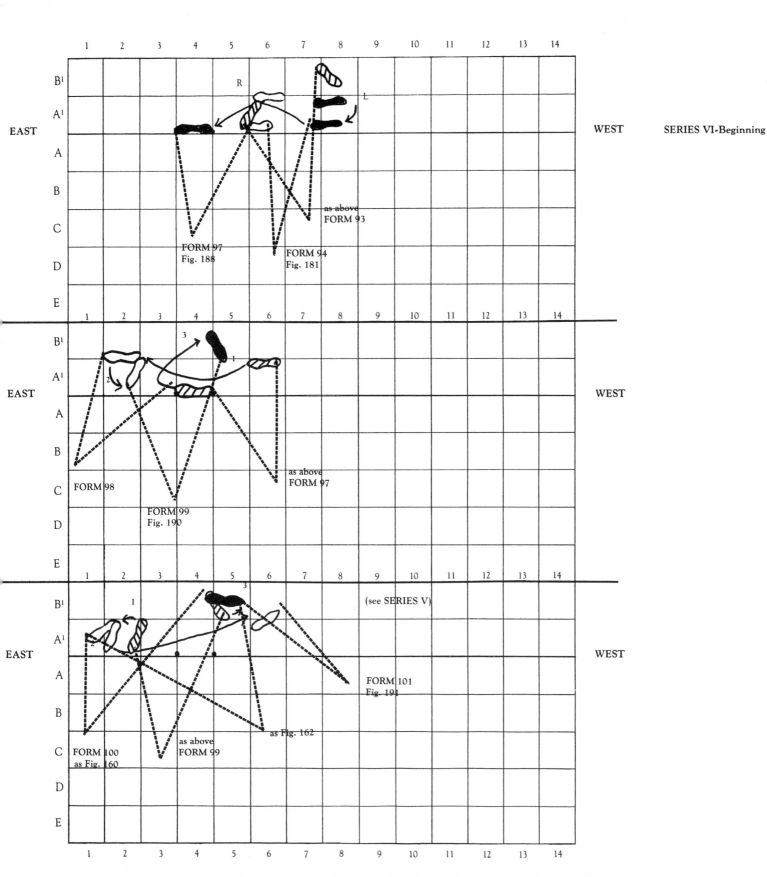

SERIES VI-Beginning

FORM 93
as above

FORM 97
Fig. 188

FORM 94
Fig. 181

FORM 98

FORM 99
Fig. 190

as above
FORM 97

FORM 100
as Fig. 160

as above
FORM 99

as Fig. 162

FORM 101
Fig. 191

(see SERIES V)

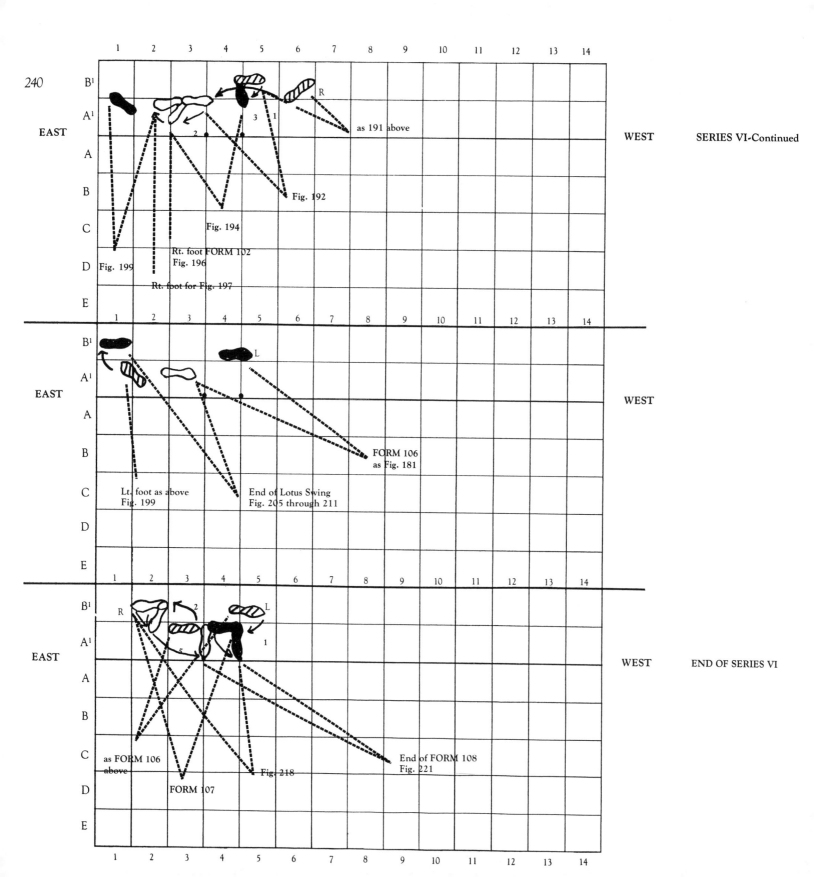

240

EAST

B¹

A¹

A

B

C

D

E

Fig. 199

Fig. 194

Rt. foot FORM 102
Fig. 196

Rt. foot for Fig. 197

Fig. 192

as 191 above

R

3  1

2

WEST    SERIES VI-Continued

EAST

B¹

A¹

A

B

C

D

E

L

FORM 106
as Fig. 181

Lt. foot as above
Fig. 199

End of Lotus Swing
Fig. 205 through 211

WEST

EAST

B¹

A¹

A

B

C

D

E

R

L

2

1

as FORM 106
above

FORM 107

Fig. 218

End of FORM 108
Fig. 221

WEST    END OF SERIES VI

# Suggested Reading

Acker, William. Tao the Hermit. London: Thames & Hudson. 1952.

Adam, Michael. Wandering in Eden. New York: Alfred A. Knopf. 1976.

Allen, C. Willard. Masters of Cathay. Shanghai: Kelly & Walsh, Ltd. 1936.

Aurobindo, Sri. The Adventure of Consciousness. Pondicherry, India: Ashram Press. 1968.

Bertherat, Therese and Carol Bernstein. The Body and Its Power. New York: Avon. 1977.

Binyon, Lawrence. The Flight of the Dragon. London: John Murray. 1959 (10th printing).

Bouquet, A. C. Sacred Books of the World. London-Baltimore: Penquin. 1914.

Bragdon, Claude. The Introduction to Yoga. New York: Alfred A. Knopf. 1933.

Bredon, Juliet. The Moon Year. Shanghai: Kelly & Walsh, Ltd. 1927.

Brunton, Paul. The Secret Path. New York: Dutton Everyman Paperback. 1935.

Bucke, Richard M., M.D. Cosmic Consciousness: A Study in the Evolution of the Human Mind. Secaucus, N.J.: The Citadel Press. 1973.

Bynner, Witter. The Way of Life. New York: John Day Company. 1944.

Capra, Fritjof. Tao of Physics. Berkeley: Shambala. 1975.

Chang, Chung-Yuan. Creativity and Taoism. New York: Julian Press, Inc. 1963.

____. Tao: A New Way of Thinking. New York: Harper and Row. 1975.

Chen, Yearning K. (Chang Kuo-Shiu, translator). T'ai-Chi Ch'üan. Shanghai: Kelly & Walsh, Ltd. 1947.

Cheng Man-Ch'ing. T'ai-Chi Ch'üan: Simplified Method of Calisthenics. Taiwan. 1962.

Ch'iu Ch'ang-Ch'an. (Timothy Richard, translator). A Mission to Heaven. Shanghai: Kelly & Walsh, Ltd. 1940.

Ch'u, Ta-Kao. Tao Te Ching. New York: Samuel Weiser. 1973.

Churchward, James. The Cosmic Forces of Mu. New York: Paperback Library, Inc. 1968.

Conger, Sarah. Letters From China. Chicago: A. C. McClure & Company. 1909.

Coomaraswamy, Ananda. The Dance of Siva. New York: The Sunrise Turn, Inc. 1918.

Cooper, J. C. Taoism: The Way of the Mystic. Northampton, England: Aquarian Press. 1972.

Crane, Louise. China in Sign and Symbol. Shanghai: Kelly & Walsh, Ltd. 1926.

Creel, Herrlee G. What is Taoism. Chicago: University of Chicago Press. 1970.

de Chardin, Teilhard. The Heart of Matter. London: A Helen & Kurt Wolff Book. 1979.

Diegh Khigh, Alx. The Eleventh Wing. Los Angeles: Nash Publishers. 1973.

Dudgeon, Dr. John, M.D., C.M. Medical Gymnastics. Tientsin, China: Journal of Peking Oriental Society. 1895.

Duyvendak, J. J. L. Tao Te Ching. London: John Murray. 1954.

Dyson, Verne. Land of the Yellow Springs. New York: Chinese Studies Press. 1937.

Edwards, E. D. The Dragon Book. London: Willard Hodge & Co., Ltd. 1919.

Feng, Gia-Fu, translator. Chuang-Tsu. New York: Vintage Books. 1974.

____, translator. Tao-Te-Ching of Lao Tsu. New York: Vintage Books. 1970.

242

Fuller, R. Buckminster. No More Second Hand God. New York: Anchor Books. 1971.

Fung Yu-Lan. (Derk Bodde, translator). A History of Chinese Philosophy. Princeton: Princeton University Press. 1952.

Giles, Lionel. The Sayings of Lao Tzu. London: John Murray. 1959 (10th printing).

____. Taoist Teachings. London: John Murray. 1912.

Giles, Herbert A., translator and annotator. Strange Stories from a Chinese Studio. Shanghai: Kelly & Walsh, Ltd. 1936.

Gitlin, Murray. Body and Mind and Their Possibilities. Philadelphia: Dorrance and Company. 1974.

Goddard, Dwight and Henry Borel. Laotzu's Tao and Wu Wei. New York: Brentano Publishers. 1919.

Goulart, Peter. The Monastery of Jade Mountain. London: John Murray. 1961

Granet, Marcel. Festivals and Songs of Ancient China. New York: E. P. Dutton and Company. 1932.

Gurdieff, G. I. Meetings with Remarkable Men. New York: E. P. Dutton and Company, Inc. 1969.

Harth, Erich. Windows on the Mind. New York: William Morrow. 1982.

Herbert, Edward. A Confucian Notebook. London: John Murray. 1950.

____. A Taoist Notebook. London: John Murray. 1955.

Hixon, Lex. Coming Home. Garden City: Anchor Books. 1978.

Hoffman, Yoel. The Sound of One Hand. New York: Basic Books. 1975.

Hou, Wai-Lu. (Wang Cheng-Chung, translator). A Short History of Chinese Philosophy. Peking: Foreign Languages Press. 1959.

Huang Wen-Shan. Fundamentals of T'ai-Chi Ch'üan. Hong Kong: South Sky Book Company. 1973.

Hughes, E. R., translator. The Art of Letters—Lu Chi's Wen Fu 302 A.D. New York: Pantheon (Bollingen Series XXIX). 1951.

Hun, Tang-Mong. The Fundamental Exercises of T'ai Chi Ch'üan (Wu Style). Singapore: Hun, Tang-Mong, Publisher, 77 Neil Road, Singapore 2. 1964.

Lau, D.C. Tao Te Ching. London: Penguin Books. 1963.

Liang, T. T. T'ai-Chi Ch'üan for Health and Self-Defense. New York: Vintage Books. 1977.

Little, Mrs. Archibald. Intimate China. London & Philadelphia: Hutchinson Co. & J. B. Lippincott Co. 1901.

Lin, Yu-Tang. The Wisdom of China. London: Michael Joseph Publisher. 1944.

Lo, Pang and Martin Inn. The Essence of T'ai Chi Ch'üan. Richmond, Calif.: North Atlantic Books. 1979.

Lu, Kuan-Yü. Taoist Yoga. New York: Samuel Weiser. 1970.

Lu, Tieh-Yuin. (Harold Shadick, translator and commentator). The Travels of Lao Tsan. Ithaca: Cornell University Press. 1952.

Luk, Charles (Lu K'uan Yu). The Secrets of Chinese Meditation. London: Rider & Company. 1964.

Ly, Hoi-Sang. Illustrious Prime Ministers: Their Ancient Manners, Customs and Philosophies. New York: Ly Hoi-Sang and Richard Alexander (privately printed). 1935.

Mason, Stephen Finney. Main Currents of Scientific Thought (Revised Edition). New York: Collier Books Science Library. 1962.

Matthiesen, Peter. The Snow Leopard. New York: The Viking Press. 1978.

McNaughton, William. The Taoist Vision. Ann Arbor, Mich.: The University of Michigan Press. 1971.

Merton, Thomas. The Way of Ch'uang Tzu. New York: New Directions. 1969.

Metzner, Ralph. Maps of Consciousness. London: Collier & Macmillan, Ltd. 1971.

Monod, Jacques. Chance and Necessity. New York: Vintage Books/Random House. 1972.

Moody, Al. I-Ching Images. Brooklyn, N.Y.: Moonbird Press. 1978.

Moore, Charles A., editor.The Chinese Mind. Honolulu: East-West Center Press & University of Hawaii Press. 1967.

Nebesky-Wojkowitz. Where the Gods are Mountains. London: Weidenfeld and Nicholson. 1956.

Needham, Joseph (FRS). Science and Civilization in China: Vol. II, History of Chinese Thought. Cambridge, England: Cambridge University Press. 1956.

Neville, Robert C. Soldier, Sage, Saint. New York: Fordham University Press. 1978.

Ornstein, Robert E. The Mind Field. New York: Pocket Books, Simon & Schuster. 1978.

Ouspensky, P. D. The Fourth Way. New York: Vintage Books. 1971.

Polos, Stephen. The Chinese Art of Healing. New York: Herder and Herder. 1971.

Rajneesh, Bhagwan Shree. When the Shoe Fits: Talks on the Stories of Chuang-Tzu. California & India: Book Graphics, Marina Del Rey, Calif. 1976.

Reymond, Lizelle. To Live Within. Garden City: Doubleday & Company. 1971.

Rieker, Hans Ulrich. Beggar Among the Dead. London: Rider & Company. 1960.

Ross, Nancy Wilson. Buddhism—The Way of Life and Thought. New York: Alfred A. Knopf. 1980.

Serrano, Miguel. The Serpent of Paradise. London: Rider & Company. 1963.

Shaffer, Edward H. Pacing the Void. Berkeley: University of California Press. 1977.

Shio, Sakanishi, translator. The Spirit of the Brush. London: John Murray. 1939.

Siren, Osvald, translator and commentator. The Chinese in the Art of Painting. New York: Schocken Books. 1953.

Siu, R. G. H. The Tao of Science. Cambridge, Mass.: M.I.T. Press. 1957.

Slaughter, Frank G., M.D. Your Body and Your Mind. New York: The New American Library. 1947.

Smith, Anthony. The Body. New York: Walker & Company. 1968.

Speiser, Werner. The Art of China. New York: Crown. 1960.

Stoddard, George. The Meaning of Intelligence. New York: Macmillan. 1943.

Sung, Z. D, The Symbols of Yi King: Vols. I & II. Shanghai: China Modern Education Company. 1934.

Sze, Mai-Mai. The Tao of Painting. New York: Pantheon (Bollingen Series XLIX). 1956.

Tseng, Chiu-Yien. The Chart of T'ai-Chi Ch'üan. Hong Kong: Union Press, Ltd. (No date).

Valery, Paul, Occasions. Princeton, N.J.: Princeton University Press. 1970.

Van der Post, Laurens. Venture to the Interior. New York. Hogarth Press, Ltd. 1952.

Van der Wetering, J. The Empty Mirror. New York: Pocket Books. 1978.

Van Gulik, R. H. Hsi K'ang and his Poetical Essay on the Lute. Tokyo: Sophia University Press & Charles E. Tuttle Company. 1968.

Verth, Ilza, translator. The Yellow Emperor's Classic of Internal Medicine. Berkeley: University of California Press. 1966.

244    Waley, Arthur. Tao the Hermit, London: Thames & Hudson, 1952.

———. Three Ways of Thought in Ancient China. New York: Doubleday Anchor Books. 1956.

———. Three Ways of Thought in Ancient China. New York: Macmillan. 1939.

Wang, Yang-Ming. (Frederich Goodrich Henke, translator). The Philosophy of Wang Yang-Ming. London-Chicago: The Open Court Publishing Company. 1916.

Watson, Burton. Early Chinese Literature. New York: Columbia University Press. 1962.

Welch, Holmes. The Parting of the Way. Boston: Beacon Press. 1957.

Werner, E. T. C. China and The Chinese. London: Sir Isaac Putnam & Sons, Ltd. 1919.

Werner, E. T. C. Myths and Legends of China. London: George Harrap & Company, Ltd. 1922.

Wieger, Leon. Taoism: The Philosophy of China. Burbank, Calif.: Ohara Publications Inc. 1976.

Wilhelm, Richard. The Secret of the Golden Flower (translated and explained). New York: Wehman Brothers. 1955.

———. I-Ching.

———, Chinese to German translator. (Cary F. Baynes is German to English translator). The I-Ching. New York: Pantheon (Bollingen Series XIX). 1950.

Wingate, Mrs. Alfred. The Golden Phoenix. London: Herbert Jenkins, Ltd. 1930.

Wright, Arthur F., editor. Studies in Chinese Thought. Chicago: University of Chicago Press. 1953.

Yu, Anthony C., translator and editor. Journey to the West. Chicago-London: University of Chicago Press. 1977.


*The following books are in Chinese:*

Ch'an, Ch'ang-Hsiang. T'ai-Chi Ch'üan Theory and Application. Taiwan: Sung Ching-Jen Publisher. 1964.

Ch'an, Chi-Fu. Comprehensive Study of Approach to T'ai-Chi Ch'üan. Taiwan: 1935.

Ch'en, Kung. Complete Story of T'ai-Chi Ch'üan. Shanghai: 1949.

Ch'u, Mien-Yu. (Introduction). T'ai-Chi Ch'üan, Exercise and Application. Peking: Department of Physical Culture. 1956.

Ho, Shao-Ju. Wu T'ang Pai (Style). Peking: Department of Physical Culture. 1963.

Hsu, Hsi-Chien. (Preface). The Practical Application of Ch'i Kung - The Therapeutic Method. Honan Province: 1962.

Hsu, Yung. Chang San-Feng's T'ai-Chi Ch'üan — Promoting Health and Longevity (Series 2). Taiwan: 1961.

Ma, Yueh-Liang and Ch'en, Chien-Ming. Wu Chien-Ch'üan's Theories on T'ai-Chi Ch'üan. Shanghai: K'an Chien Books. 1935 and 1948.

Sheng, Chia-Ch'eng and Ku, Liu-Hsing. T'ai-Chi Ch'üan Chen Style (Series one). Peking: Department of Physical Culture. 1963.

Ts'ai, Ho-Peng. T'ai-Chi Ch'üan, Yang style. Hong Kong: 1956.

T'ang, Hao. Roots of T'ai-Chi Ch'üan. Hong Kong: 1935.

Tung, Ying-Chieh. T'ai-Chi Ch'üan System — Yang Style. Hong Kong: 1964.